STARING AT THE PARK

WRITING LIVES

Ethnographic Narratives

Series Editors:

Arthur P. Bochner & Carolyn Ellis

University of South Florida

Writing Lives: Ethnographic Narratives publishes narrative representations of qualitative research projects. The series editors seek manuscripts that blur the boundaries between humanities and social sciences. We encourage novel and evocative forms of expressing concrete lived experience, including autoethnographic, literary, poetic, artistic, visual, performative, critical, multi-voiced, conversational, and co-constructed representations. We are interested in ethnographic narratives that depict local stories; employ literary modes of scene setting, dialogue, character development, and unfolding action; and include the author's critical reflections on the research and writing process, such as research ethics, alternative modes of inquiry and representation, reflexivity, and evocative storytelling. Proposals and manuscripts should be directed to abochner@cas.usf.edu

Volumes in this series:

1 *Erotic Mentoring: Women's Transformations in the University*, Janice Hocker Rushing
2 *Intimate Colonialism: Head, Heart, and Body in West African Development Work*, Laurie L. Charlés
3 *Last Writes: A Daybook for a Dying Friend*, Laurel Richardson
4 *A Trickster in Tweed: The Quest for Quality in a Faculty Life*, Thomas F. Frentz
5 *Guyana Diaries: Women's Lives Across Difference*, Kimberly D. Nettles
6 *Writing Qualitative Inquiry: Selves, Stories and the New Politics of Academic Success*, H. L. Goodall, Jr.
7 *Accidental Ethnography: An Inquiry into Family Secrecy*, Christopher N. Poulos
8 *Revision: Autoethnographic Reflections on Life and Work*, Carolyn Ellis
9 *Leaning: A Poetics of Personal Relations*, Ronald J. Pelias
10 *Narrating the Closet: An Autoethnography of Same-Sex Attraction*, Tony E Adams
11 *Life After Leaving: The Remains of Spousal Abuse*, Sophie Tamas
12 *Playing with Purpose: Adventures in Performative Social Science*, Mary M. Gergen and Kenneth J. Gergen
13 *Critical Autoethnography: Intersecting Cultural Identities in Everyday Life*, Robyn M. Boylorn and Mark P. Orbe
14 *Coming to Narrative: A Personal History of Paradigm Change in the Human Sciences*, Arthur P. Bochner
15 *Transcribing Silence: Culture, Relationships, and Communication*, Kristine L. Muñoz
16 *Staring at the Park: A Poetic Autoethnographic Inquiry*, Jane Speedy

STARING AT THE PARK

A Poetic Autoethnographic Inquiry

Jane Speedy

Routledge
Taylor & Francis Group
LONDON AND NEW YORK

First published 2015 by Left Coast Press, Inc.

Published 2016 by Routledge
2 Park Square, Milton Park, Abingdon, Oxon OX14 4RN
711 Third Avenue, New York, NY 10017, USA

Routledge is an imprint of the Taylor & Francis Group, an informa business

Library of Congress Cataloging-in-Publication Data

Speedy, Jane, 1954-
Staring at a park : a poetic autoethnographic inquiry / Jane Speedy, Walnut Creek, California.
pages cm. — (Writing lives : ethnographic narratives ; 16)
Includes bibliographical references.
ISBN 978-1-62958-122-4 (hardback : alk. paper)—ISBN 978-1-62958-124-8 (institutional eBook)—ISBN 978-1-62958-125-5 (consumer eBook)
1. Speedy, Jane, 1954- 2. Cerebrovascular disease—Patients—United States—Biography. 3. Cerebrovascular disease—Patients—Rehabilitation. 4. Parks—Psychological aspects. 5. Visualization—Therapeutic use. I. Title.
RC388.5.S65 2015
362.196'810092—dc23
[B]

2015004494

ISBN-13: 978-1-62958-122-4 (hbk)
ISBN-13: 978-1-62958-123-1 (pbk)

Contents

List of illustrations **7**

Acknowledgments **8**

Guide to textual style and protocols **9**

Foreword: Staring with Jane **10**
Ken Gale and Jonathan Wyatt

Introduction **13**
How and why I wrote this book

First plateau **17**
I wrote this book three times/txt

Second plateau **45**
A process of writing developed eventually or at least a method of/pdf

Third plateau **93**
We rattled through wrought iron gates/doc

Fourth plateau **117**
Early morning silence/docx

Fifth plateau **139**
Park haiku/winged/docx

Sixth plateau **159**
Epilogue/solitude is what I live with a constant lack of/txt

Notes **177**

References **179**

About the author **184**

For Sarah and Carter

List of Illustrations

First plateau	*horse chestnut* **17**
	spring trees **34**
	trees in conversation **34**
	summer trees **39**
	autumn trees **39**
	more trees in conversation **43**
Second plateau	*spring in the park* **45**
	summer in the park **54**
	autumn in the park **54**
	winter in the park **67**
	horse chestnut again **67**
	angel from mars **76**
Third plateau	*horse chestnut and me – entanglement* **93**
	trails of tape **103**
	whispering bats **103**
	trails of tape 2 **105**
	residual traces in the grass **105**
	fox tracks in the snow **115**
Fourth plateau	*residual traces in the grass 2* **117**
	tracks through the park **127**
	coffin trail to baddock woods **127**
	non-human tracks **134**
	more non-human tracks **134**
	night branches **137**
Fifth plateau	*night flight* **139**
	trails **143**
	window on the park **143**
	kantha shawl **153**
	multiple kantha shawls **153**
	the winged creature's cloak **156**
Sixth plateau	*through the window* **159**
	fragmented views **167**
	early morning in the park **167**
	paths remember people **170**
	splintered pathway **170**
	six-headed serpent **175**

Acknowledgments

I would like to thank the friends and colleagues who read and commented on earlier versions of this text, in particular: Sue Porter, Jonathan Wyatt, Ken Gale, Artemis Sakellariadis, Ann Rippin, Goya Wilson Vasquez, Bubukee Pyrsou, and Donna Kemp. I also owe thanks to my companions at the 2013 Hawkswood College writing retreat where this project started, including: Jo Kirby, Margaret Page, Maud Perrier, Jeannie Wright, Marina Malthouse and Sarah Hall. And to the 'Narrative Open Space' members in the Graduate School of Education, where I first presented this work, including: Jelena Nolan-Miljevic, Prue Bramwell-Davies, Peggy Styles, Malcolm Reed, and Jan Filer. I also owe gratitude and thanks to those who have encouraged me to pursue a late trajectory as a visual artist, including Esme Clutterbuck, Davina Kirkpatrick, Tessa Wyatt, and Sue Tate. This work also owes a huge debt to the Canadian classics scholar and poet, Ann Carson, whom I have never met, but whose work casts both a deep shadow and several blinding shards of light throughout my book.

This is the point where I start to thank everybody I have ever met in my life and everywhere I have ever been, all of whom have left residual traces of those meetings and those landscapes for me to gather up and weave somewhere into this work, but I think I'll stop now, and just end by thanking Mitch, Art, and Carolyn before things get really out of hand and I begin to include the spectral splinters of my own future. Mitch Allen of the Left Coast Press, Inc., and Art Bochner and Carolyn Ellis, editors of the *Writing Lives: Ethnographic Narratives* series have between them taken the risk of publishing this qwerky, beautiful little book by a writer from the 'wrong side of the pond' at a time when a much larger, glossier European publishing house pronounced it 'economically unviable', which just goes to show that there are multiple versions of viability in this life. I am still not sure if I wrote this book, or produced it, or 'curated' it. In any case, here it is.

Guide to textual style and protocols

Life is made up of fragments.
We never have all the pieces
cannot ever see the whole

Fragments get garbled, misunderstood
and distorted

taken out of sequence

They make up life.

(Nobbs, 2011, p. 3)

This book is written in narrow strips or fragments of text, most of which contain embedded citations in the usual style of academic prose. This text is also interwoven with images and text boxes or postcards that are placed at juxtapositions, adjacent to the flow of the main text. The postcards bordered with a thin black line are written by the author and the grey-filled postcards (like this one from Nobbs) are quotations from other people's work.

These text boxes or postcards contain writings (whether by the author or another writer) that engage with, and overlap, the main flow of the text: these 'samples' from other refrains or themes may be spliced into this text, but may equally fit onto another page of this book, or indeed, into another text altogether. In this way, to quote Benjamin (1927/1999, p. 871), 'the rags, the refuse – these I will not inventory but allow, in the only way possible, to come into their own: by making use of them'.

Foreword
Staring with Jane

Ken Gale and Jonathan Wyatt

On 21 July 2014, we received an email from Jane, which read:

> Feels like a rave from the grave.... writing an e-mail to my 'two boys'.... I was wondering whether I could persuade/entice/seduce you two into writing a foreword for my 'staring at the park' book...I should have the final first draft ready next month for you to read..... and the book (including foreword) needs to be oven ready by mid October. I was thinking of which person to ask to do this .... and then I remembered that I was mid-writing a foreword for your 'Writing Touches' book, when I had a stroke....so I jettisoned the 'a person' notion... in favour of turning the tables.... would you two conjointly like to write my foreword? I'd really like that.... go on, you'd make an old tart very happy....

We agreed, of course. Delighted, honoured, excited; simultaneously amused and moved by Jane's invitation. We had known Jane was working on this text, we had seen early drafts of some chapters, and enjoyed the iPad pictures that Jane had been creating. Yet somehow the news we received from her, a few weeks before this email, that the book was almost ready and accepted by Left Coast Press, seemed sudden. Jane is always full of surprises. Jane is a surprise.

So we said yes, then separately but together began to write and to send each other our thoughts, riffing off – a key metaphor of Jane's in this book – each other and off our reading of Jane's wonderful work. Ken began, then a few weeks' gap while Jonathan was away, then Ken again.

Starring at the Park: A Poetic Autoethnographic Inquiry, Jane Speedy, 10–12.

Ken, 19 August

Ron Bogue says:

> The notion of 'overflight' or *survol*, requires special attention. The word *survol* designates the act of flying over the ground in an airplane, and by extension, the act of rapidly scanning a page with the eyes. Deleuze and Guattari take the idea of *survol* as developed here by Raymond Ruyer, who identifies this 'overflight' with the primary consciousness of all living forms. (2003, p.172)

Flying, scanning, soaring, dipping, taking it all in and not, thinking about barn owls' eyes, thinking about buzzards, all the way up there, looking all the way down here. 'Did you see that mouse scratch its nose?' I didn't, the buzzard did, ergo 'the primary consciousness of all living forms'.

Foreword can be starting in the middle, flying and scanning and kind of digesting what you have seen so far and then thinking whether to zoom in and pounce or whether to wait for another thermal and do some more sky dancing before slow, slow, quick, quick, slowing it into the next stage of the refrain.

I have been flying and skimming with Jane's writing this morning: it's lovely. It's all about becoming, it's all about difference within and not between: every time Jane repeats she is different and that is the joy of this writing. It never sits still; 'the primary consciousness of all living forms' is always shifting coming alive and never ending...

Jonathan, 16 September

Many weeks later. So much since then, since flying with Ken's words over Jane's, seeing them from that distance, high up, catching sight, catching sound, catching alight. Flown. Time has. Weeks of a life needing to be lived on the ground, eyes down, lifting feet step by step, unable to see the wood from the knees.

But all the while I remembered; remembered *survol*, remembered Jane, remembered this book.

Staring at the Park is a work of art. When she woke from her stroke –

> (Stop: 'woke'? Too benign, as if Jane had been for a peaceful afternoon nap. When Jane 'came to'? 'Re-emerged'? 'Re-turned'? None of these works. It's the prefix. 'Re-': the same again; is back. No. Not so. Not for Jane. Not for any of us. Ever.
>
> Try again:

When Jane surfaced – yes? Better. Surfaced from drowning. The danger, the risk, implicit. The loss of control.)

So: When Jane surfaced, she asked for poetry. Not for water. Not for Sarah, or Carter. She didn't ask what the time was, what day it was, what happened, where she was, who she was. She asked for poetry, desperate to know: 'Language would be a terrible, unimaginable loss', she writes.

This book is evidence that she still has it. And some. I leave the ground on her poetry, taking flight again with her, with this book. Take flight on her fractured lines. Take flight on her ruptured, suturing words through the landscape of her stroke and its aftermath. Jane talks of 'staring'; she invites us into 'a practice of staring: staring that leads to writing and drawing'. It sounds as if such a practice might be quiet, passive – and as if creating the book were these for her – but it is staring as *action*: as dance, as protest, as embrace, as struggle, as despair, as anger; staring as noise, as music, as art. Staring as love. As loss. As *survol.*

I am in wonder here. I am at home looking up from our Edinburgh basement flat onto the pavement above. Through the squares of our kitchen sash window I see only the lower legs of people walking past, glimpses of cars, the sun on the sandstone walls of the tenements across the road. I am learning to stare.

Ken, 28 September

There seem to be many filmic resonances between our sense of becoming with Jane as she stared, and continues to stare, into her park and the rich imagery and vibrant narratives of Wim Wender's film *Wings of Desire*. It feels as if, as in Wender's film, there are invisible, undying angels floating in, through and above Jane's staring. Her writing in this book is full of what Deleuze might describe as a productive desire, a form of desire that works to heal and comfort and that refuses to die. On awakening and flying back into this waking world, just as Wender's angel becomes an earthly angel, Jane, in asking for poetry, knew that the loss of language would be unbearable. Jane's writing here not only relishes the urgent sensual and sensory beauty of living in the world it works to produce, enrich and fulfill through its presence on these pages. There is a strong sense in reading Jane's book that we are able to soar with her and, in so doing, are able, like the angel in the film becoming in human life, to live a life of colour, intense joy and deep, sensual pleasure and love.

Introduction
How and why I wrote this book

After the stroke life became increasingly poetic, written in snatches. I found poems in fragments of conversation as people passed by my hospital bed. These fragments could have been for or about me or just caught up in the underpinning and scaffolding of my life, in passing. There was yet more poetry trapped within the clanking of ambulances and the passing of trolleys and equipment. There were shredded haiku between the blinds of hospital kitchens and corridors. My friends brought me books of poetry, which offered shorter, cleaner and sharper excursions into other worlds than either novels, which were too long, or learned medical papers about strokes, which were too boring. The economy and amplification that poetry brought into my life was something I could make sense of, and digest between medical/ hospital/social events....

And so it seemed as though I listened to the world around me as if at a recital or performance, and this book became a poetic and performative inquiry into my fragmented, disjointed life. I began to realize, through this amplified version, that all of life is disjointed and fragmented and that the linear narrative I had been living was just a conceit. I read all the 'stroke survivor's narratives' I could get my hands on, but despaired at the neatness of the endings and coherence of the stories. Was I the only person whose life seemed to have been chopped up by this? I began again to realize that everybody is disabled and that the perfection of able bodies was another conceit: I began to view able bodiedness as a 'regime of truth'. We are all imperfect and all our work/actions/lives are embodied. I read today in the newspaper of the invention of a decelerator helmet that could be used with stroke survivors in hospital (Buchan, 2014). My world was already decelerated, perhaps I could use such a helmet to decelerate the rest. In hospital I was surrounded by elderly women with lives in accelerated tatters. In hospital things just happen to you. Deceleration is required. There is

Starring at the Park: A Poetic Autoethnographic Inquiry, Jane Speedy, 13–16.

no control. Shards of my experience were left, littered and interrupted all over the hospital. Indeed, this whole 'becoming/being in hospital' experience was a giant interruption to life as I had intended to live it.

In hospital I took copious notes, but even those notes, when I read them back to myself on returning home, held a chaotic/poetic echo. I sat in my bedroom at home, reading my notes, staring out at the park. I began to write this book on the iPad I had bought myself, but even then, it could not write itself into a neatly ended and coherent whole. It came out in fragments, some days in shards of poetry, some days in images. My method was to look out of my bedroom window and record what I was thinking, feeling, doing, hearing and seeing. I also made notes on the various books I had taken up into the bedroom. This was precarious listening and note-taking indeed.

The stories of this experience are re-presented in this book in the form of layers of fragmented poetic text and image. This is my embodied/visceral/textual resistance to narrative coherence and my means of bringing experience to life. These stories are re-presented, but not represented here. This text tentatively negotiates an auto-ethnographic position, offering a facsimile or tattered palimpsest, alongside the ruined life narrative. I cannot represent, or even pretend to understand, my experience, but nonetheless I long to, and am compelled to try to communicate/perform and approximate the stutterings, intensities, moods and flavours (see Gale, 2014) of this life as lived. I am propelled by an ethic of living my life and of being alive, even, despite and perhaps because of these times of contested selves, into giving an account of my 'self' (Butler, 2005). In other words, I am giving an account of this life as an act of homage or gratitude. I am so glad that I am not dead.

I have had great difficulty in discerning the borders and edges that can disentangle 'my life' from its surroundings, why would I even begin to try to do that? But I have found the poetic and visual forms of representation set down here to bring that process of (dis)entanglement and contestation to life and to the fore.

I was disappointed with the stroke survivor narratives I came across, mostly written by young men, and I partly wrote this text for myself and partly for Maud, Mabel, Ivy, Elsie and the other flower girls in the stroke ward: the many confused and disoriented elderly people I met and spent time with in hospital. I wrote this book against the grain of the more triumphalist, coherent, archetypically 'male' mountain-climbing survivor narratives that I was given to read. I wanted to privilege confusion and incoherence and old age and to express a resistance to the pioneering, more youthful myths that made coherent and linear sense of it all.

If I had not had a stroke in my late 50s, my life would never have been thrown up against the lives of Mabel and Ivy and Elsie, and the other, often confused, elderly women I was in hospital with. Some of them were grandmothers, still others had been nuns, yet others had been the champion cyclists of their day, and I spent hours exchanging stories with them. I knew their fragmentations as they knew mine. We all lived in fear of the same staff nurse when she came to 'aspirate' us. Having known these women, however, I now no longer fear old age. This is my story, not theirs, but it has been written, in many senses, in their company.

The names and events in this book have been fictionalised, the places and spaces around Bristol and my own life events have not. This book does not come with an instruction manual. It is up to you how or whether you read it and which bits you skim over, but it does come with this introduction, which goes some way to explain how and why I wrote it in the way I did. There are other sections scattered throughout this text where I add to this explication, particularly throughout 'plateau one' (after Deleuze and Guattari, 1987), where I outline the history of the writing and drawing process as it changed over time, and in 'plateau two' where I explain my emerging method of representing a life in fragments and its relationship with the work of Carson (1999, 2012) and Finkel (2014). Carson and Finkel make interesting mentors: Carson is a classics scholar and contemporary poet and Finkel an archaeologist and writer of children's fiction. Finkel has not yet combined, overlapped and confused his academic and literary writings as I have tried to do here, although sediments and traces always lurk and seep. Indeed, Carson's writing includes and blends poetry, essay, prose, criticism, translation, dramatic dialogue, fiction, and non-fiction.

Not unlike Benjamin's 'arcades project' the method of constructing this book was that the pieces formed a montage or layered account of my life, spread out between passages of text from various books, papers and poems, and images of the park, and of what I saw and heard of 'the rags, the refuse – these I will not inventory but allow, in the only way possible, to come into their own: by making use of them'(Benjamin, 1999, p. iN1a7). Unlike Benjamin's magnum opus, this project is deliberately and explicitly small, partial, contingent and particular and took only three years, not thirteen, to come to a loosely unraveling, unfinished halt. I was inquiring solely into the soundscapes and landscapes outside my window, not into the state of the world, although implicitly they reflect each other. These were the images that I was setting down on my iPad, in juxtaposition with my thoughts, feelings, ways of looking, everyday life events, and the books and papers I had access to. These sources I did not so much 'plug into' in the way that Jackson and Mazzei (2013), after Deleuze and Guattari (1987), describe. My method, as well as staring, was more that of 'riffing off'. Indeed, I prefer the less mechanistic 'riffing off' metaphor, with its origins in jazz improvisations and repeated melodic refrains, perhaps with a slight change of key. This book riffs off Anne Carson's (1999) poetry and David Hockney's (2012) iPad paintings in the ways that other researchers tend to privilege a riffing off or improvisation taken from theoretical writings and social science texts. This text is not, then, so much an effort towards a 'doubled science' (Lather, 2007) as towards an arts-based method whereby I give an account of myself in time, place and space, albeit uncertainly, without really knowing what I am doing or where I am going. Like Lather (2007) I am setting out to get myself lost. The text forms an assemblage. Multiplicities collide, rather than congeal into coherence. I have not got there. This work is not finished, there is no 'final arrival', whereby the 'tripartite division' 'between a field of reality (the world) and a field of representation (the book) and a field of subjectivity (the author)' (Jackson & Mazzei, 2013, p. 263) combines. This text is temporary, and I temporarily invite you in. Later we can change it.

As a poetic text this book is informed by a qualitative research tradition that has an interdisciplinary wealth of practitioners all pushing in the same direction, proclaiming poetic texts as relevant forms of representation for research interviews and conversations (Richardson, 1997, 2001), which also capture/encapsulate the vitality required in life writing (Etherington, 2004; Prendergast, 2009; West, 2012). In presenting my text in this way, I lean heavily on the shoulders of those who have gone before me and share their hopes for an accessible way into a web of complex, confusing, contradictory narratives and a 'magnified sense' (Prendergast, 2009, p. xi) of experience. I share their belief that poetic/arts-informed representation might be 'more heartfelt, more concentrated, more distilled' (Piirto, 2012, p. 435) than more prosaic representations and hope that my use of poetic text troubles the falseness of the representation/reality binary. I am offering this incomplete, uncertain text, thinking with and riffing off post-human and feminist theory, contemporary poetry and visual inquiry, together with a plethora of pictures, papers and postcards purloined along the way. Walter Benjamin (1999), with his enormous cultural vision and two good legs, was a *flaneur*: a master of the art of strolling. I refrain from too much strolling in my park. I prefer flying. But for now, from my bedroom eyrie, I am inviting you into a practice of staring: a precarious staring in multiple directions and ways that leads, in this instance, to writing and drawing. I am inviting you to join with me in staring at the park.

First plateau

I wrote this book three times/txt

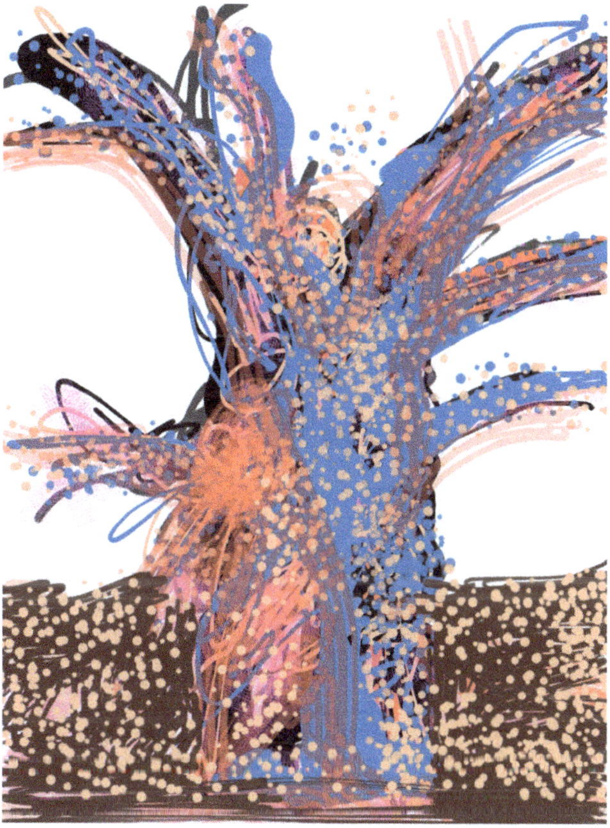

horse chestnut

Staring at the Park: A Poetic Autoethnographic Inquiry, Jane Speedy, 17–43.

This…contains a story and several other things. The other things might be connected with the story, or they might not; they might be connected to stories that haven't appeared yet. It's not easy to tell. It's easy to imagine how they might have turned up though. The world is full of things like that: old post cards, theatre programmes, leaflets about bomb-proofing your cellar … All these tattered old bits and pieces have a history and a meaning. A group of them together can seem like traces…

(Pullman, 2003, p. i)

I WROTE THIS BOOK THREE TIMES. It was, to misquote my dear friend and mentor Cathy Riessman[1] a thrice-told tale. In its first incarnation this inquiry was firmly divided into three separate accounts of the park: an ethnographic study of the park environment and the people who passed through it; a murder mystery surrounding the body found in the paddling pool in the children's park; and an excerpt from the life story of the author, a former professor of education and the director of a narrative research centre at the university of Bristol whose life had taken an unexpected turn after she had suffered a severe stroke and found herself grounded from her academic career, spending a lot of her days sitting in the first floor bedroom of her house overlooking the park, staring out of the window.

It was only on rereading these narratives alongside each other that I realised that all three pieces of work centred on and had in a sense emerged from the park opposite my house, and that my primary research and storytelling method in all three instances was 'staring into the space in front of me'. These inquiries were interconnected. They had started life as ventures into three separate genres: ethnography, fiction and life story. They had been religiously and methodically separated into different writing styles and different spaces in my life, my mind and on my computer. But together they constituted a poetics of the park.

In its second incarnation this inquiry became four intertwined and parallel narrative accounts emerging from the same space: one work of fiction; one piece of social ethnographic research and one auto-ethnographic tale; each interspersed with iPad paintings of the park, each narrative gradually leaking and spilling over its genre boundaries into the other. I set all this work out in a 'Dropbox'[2] folder on the web – the three written narratives running through the text in a linear parallel. And there they sat. Something was wrong with the very manicured sense of time and memory surfacing in this work when it was laid out in its neatly labelled "docx" folders; something about the coherence and chronological tidiness of these carefully bordered (albeit leaking) narratives jarred with my understanding. I was somehow divorcing imagination, scholarly inquiry and everyday life from each other and constructing them as separate categories of experience, placing them in separate (docx) folders.

In its third incarnation I told this story again as a conjointly constructed, narrative; built with shards of imagined, lived and observed experience, each crashing in on the other. This thrice-told tale (imagined, researched and lived) of meandering through the shared territory of the park opposite my house, assimilated interlocking fragments of story and image from my accumulated experience of staring out of my first floor bedroom bay window into the park. This was not an ethnography of the park, but an ethnography only of that which could be seen, envisaged or imagined from my bedroom window. fictional accounts of the life of the park and accounts of the life of the writer were no longer separated out into stories disconnected from ethnographic observations. I was, in any case, a participant observer only in so far as I could observe life in the corner of St Andrews park at the intersection between Maurice road and Leopold road, just down the park below the paddling pool in the children's park (my house is on Leopold road, right on this corner) and only in so far as I could walk with my stick slowly up to the corner and/or trundle in my powered wheelchair up to the post office on Derby Road to purchase a copy of the Guardian newspaper. These horizons may seem limited, but my view includes the contents of a mind well stocked with literary and scholarly texts; a lifetime informed by practices as a narrative inquirer and therapist and a vivid and well-stocked imagination, as well as actual and virtual access to the University of Bristol library services and all the internet access and painting and drawing apps that an iPad has to offer. It is a neurological curiosity that my mind can no longer remember how to wave my left hand or bend my left knee, but my worldview is as informed as it ever was by Mark Freeman's[3] conceptualisations of autobiographical, narrative, and chronological time; Gaston Bachelard's (1994) theories of a human 'poetics of space' and Wendy Faris's (2004) scholarly accounts of magical realism as post-colonial critique. The 'five rhythms dancer'[4] – has been stopped in her tracks, but the 'narrative scholar' continues/ where we have no histories, we honour our ancestors, like Toni Morrison (1987), by imagining their lives and thence our own/those neat and coherent and always triumphant post-stroke stories I have come across (Bolte-Taylor, 2009; Klein, 1998; McCrum, 1998)[5] left my disjointed existence uncharted, unstoried and unheard. Perhaps I have no ancestors or kindred spirits?/ And then I remember Mabel and Ivy in the stroke ward/Or was it Marlene and Iris?/ and the desire expressed towards them and towards us all by the medical profession to 'get back to normal'. Let us not, then, speak in honour or praise of the chaos and incoherence that those of us left behind and alive are left with/let us not imagine what those different (decelerated?) lives and stories might be/shall we speak of walking and talking and of 'getting back to normal'?/ I had always replied to the medical profession that I was still searching for my new 'normal'/I still am/ the journalist, Andrew Marr[6] had a very similar stroke to mine about a year later/he too had charted his life before and after his stroke with an iPad and he too had always made sense of his world through drawing and writing / he, perhaps wisely, tells us very little about his stroke, other than not having any idea himself of how ill he was and presumably since he is now back doing his old job, he has achieved his new normal/

THIS BOOK HAS BEEN WRITTEN AND DRAWN AS IF TORN INTO SHREDS/ that fit together somehow/and together/ make up the parts that shape my world and write my life/inner and outer geographies and territories /pieces of writing and iPad paintings /interrupted and renamed as 'docx' or 'jpeg' on my computer/ imaginings images readings and knowledge/ garnered on a journey through a dense fog that has sustained itself no matter what weather conditions were blowing about in the park/ or in my densely fogged mind/ and clung to the corners/sometimes taking over my soul completely/ this text mirrors experience in both form and content/ no matter whether docx/jpeg/ png or txt/ it will not be an easy read/or ride/ my purpose is to show you what life has been like for me these past two years/ post-the-stroke/ which struck on November 16th 2011/I am writing this two years later/ and I feel very alive/

Riffing off in the jazz improvisation sense, rather than plugging in the machinic sense opens the door to 'sampling' – another contemporary musical metaphor – and thus this text is scattered with grey text boxes – samples from other texts that engage with my work/ instead of/ as well as / the carefully placed and embedded citations of traditional academic prose/ my text includes multiple samples from adjacent works – juxtapositioned temporarily alongside my writing and images. Juxtapositions lead like thresholds, only placed on corners. This work is peppered with thresholds – open doorways to other territories but the thresholds are throughways – straightforward transactions – textbox juxtapositions are like thresholds deliberately and obscurely placed around corners where no obvious point of entry or opening can be discerned...

A similar scattering of boxes has occurred within my own writing – postcards full of writing that could belong somewhere in this text/ wherein they have fallen/ been placed /they might equally belong somewhere else in the world/ they might have slipped into the envelope alongside the gas bill or into a little pile on the mantelpiece together with invitations to funerals and weddings/ such juxtapositions come in a scattering of textboxes – my own writing is like this – in a box surrounded, like funeral invitations by a thin black line..., writing by other authors is in white font on a grey background.

CARLY WAS THE YUMMIEST OF THE MUMMIES/HER LITTLE OTTO THE CHUBBIEST, most organically fed of the park babies/her jogging gear in navy and lime green with matching socks and trainers/ matched the livery of little Otto's superbuggy/ lime and navy are this year's colours/ little Otto sat sedately in a grand three-wheeler range-rover buggy manufactured from locally sourced ingredients/ Carly married Justin straight after Uni/they both went into corporate law, but Carly quit when she fell pregnant/not the kind of job that suits new parents /corporate law/ she couldn't cope with the all-nighters /as well as Otto's unpredictability/

IT IS RANDOM/ THIS WHO GETS WRITTEN OR DRAWN IN AND WHO GETS WRITTEN OR DRAWN OUT of the text/image business/ the episode with the newts in the pond at the Maurice road entrance below the bowling green for instance / that got scrapped from this version /as did the whole eco-warrior park narrative/ writing in and writing out of history/ it has happened to whole genders before/ and has depended throughout history on who found and translated the original stories and on the order in which the fragments of manuscript were placed/ in the newspaper today, Irving Finkel (2014) the curator of the clay tablets collection in the British museum[7] told again the story of Noah and his ark full of animals/ this time he did not tell the Judeo-Christian story, but the preceding Mesopotamian and Babylonian versions that he had translated from his clay tablets, telling us of a round ark/ and today it is my editing that shapes these park chronicles of people criss-crossing and getting murdered/this leaves out those whose trajectories that circumnavigate my corner of the park /I leave out what I cannot see or even imagine/ I include rumours of ferrets, but not of newts / some lives are written in/ some trees are finger painted/others not/

I SUSPECT THAT THIS IS AN ACCOUNT OF A MORE ACUTELY EXPERIENCED VERSION OF WHAT IT MEANS TO BE HUMAN THAN most of us have in our everyday lives/ (or maybe this is just what happens when you cut an experienced narrative inquirer adrift from her scholarly moorings and leave her with enough space to stare into /searching for meaning in a small corner/amongst myriad fragments/ that may be connected /or they may not/ but may simply have been blown in together on the wind off the Atlantic ocean) / humans make stories and paint pictures which in turn make meanings, where, perhaps, there is in 'reality' only weather (albeit gale force at times)/

LAST NIGHT THERE WAS THUNDER AND LIGHTENING. I OPENED THE BLINDS AND WATCHED THE LIGHTENING SHEETING DOWN INTO THE PARK. THE SKY WAS IN FULL FLOW AND THE TREES WERE

CREAKING/Under the avenue of limes / I caught sight of a hooded figure, scampering about between the trees/ a fairy perhaps? The thunder was some miles away/ the lightening falling down in sleek sheets through attic windows/ scorching around the room/then leaching out down the roof/dropping off molten into the garden/charred holes in the deck my only proof/

THE ORDINARY AND EVERYDAY ARE MY LUXURIES/NOW my life has gone into extra time/your dark pink hanging candelabra stare through the window/ our friendship an unexpected bonus/ these horse chestnuts, captured and surrounded by the city/as urban as I am/they spill their seeds and fruit onto concrete pathways and the seasons pass them by every bit as much as I pass them by/their branches gaze through the bedroom windows of Victorian houses/

This writing was inscribed on the park /great swathes of words tattooed across the ground/carved into tree trunks/littering the pathways/the drawings meanwhile were evoked by the trees/drawn out of the author through the material efficacy of the environment that she was staring at/the horse chestnut/ in particular/became starer to her staree /the agency of the horse chestnut, and of all the trees, in drawing out these images/was extraordinary at first/until this process of staring at/drawing/ othering or writing into the park became a daily practice/It started with an iPad and the drawing/first up there was always a drawing/the park was drawing on the author/ she was writing then on the trees/

The project become a semi-collaborative venture – not collaborative with other people, but a collaboration with trees and pathways and between different modalities/ together with a process of drawing out what could be seen in/by the park/different views of the same landscape and a melding of different ways of seeing (and becoming) this space.

THIS IS NOT A STROKE SURVIVOR'S NARRATIVE, written with other stroke survivors in mind – this is an account written against the grain of such accounts and realities, most of which, however well written, seem to leave out any disjunctures within the world:

> inappropriate peals of laughter/ disastrous bladder control/and ignore the blank spaces staring at the floor/in between rational moments of life narrative as if they were uninhabited by the author/they paper over the blank days with coherent thoughts and credible inhabitants (Bolte-Taylor, 2009; McCrum, 1998)

I am not with them in this 'normalising'. I am with Jeanette Winterson (2004, p. 196), who says: 'I do not accept that life has an ordinary shape, or that there is anything ordinary about life at all. We make it ordinary, but it is not'.

Nor am I with Molly Andrews (2014) who has just produced a book in this manner of 'making ordinary', as I am writing, entitled: '*Narrative imagination and everyday life*', thus engendering a distinct border between categories and narratives imagined and categories and narratives of the every day and, indeed, between imagination and life.

I, and this book, alongside Walter Benjamin with his anticipation of dream, image and imagination as new means of inquiring (1999, pp.

192–198), inhabit these border territories, these spaces where lives imagined and ordinary; everyday and extraordinary, overlap each other in meaning, shape size and space, dancing along the way on glass feet that splinter into a thousand shards and spill across our lives.

WHEN I WAS IN HOSPITAL ARTEMI SENT ME A BOXED SET of the first two series of Downton Abbey (Fellowes, 2010–present)/ I could follow the plot day after day/ I could manage this and start again where I had left off the night before/whereas books or at least novels, totally eluded me/For the most part in hospital I read poetry and listened to music/ Poetry /Short interludes with intimate, beautiful language and an economy and density of expression that took me out into different spaces/ Sarah found me a new poet – Tomas Transtroemer, of whom I had never heard /despite his winning that year's Nobel prize for literature for 'giving us fresh access to reality' (Astley, 2011) / I discovered also that eleven years previously he had suffered a stroke / perhaps that was partly why his sharp, intense, visual poetry spoke so keenly to and for me?/Perhaps he too saw the world with fresh eyes or perhaps his eyes had always been held so widely open to his world? / Certainly his earlier poems had an equally fresh translucent quality/I was in a busy crowded inner city hospital ward and his poems took me to out into the quiet of Scandanavian forests:

> *one can go slowly on skis in the winter sun,*
>
> *through brush where a few leaves hang on.*
>
> *They resemble pages torn from old telephone directories.*
>
> (Transtroemer, *After a Death,* 1997)

HAZEL BROUGHT ME CAROL ANN DUFFY'S 'THE BEES' (2011). The hardcover copy was a gorgeous little book to hold in my hand whilst I was 'the human bee' in my cell in the hospital where 'I could not fly and I made no honey'

> So that was my working 1ife as a bee,
> till my eyesight blurred,
> my hand was a trembling bird
> in the leaves,
> the bones of my fingers thinner than wands.
> And when they retired me,
> I had my wine from the silent vines,
> and I'd known love,
> and I'd saved some money –
> but I could not fly and I made no
> honey.
>
> (Carol Ann Duffy, 2011)

poetry could be put down and the books picked up again in the short/ interrupted shots of time I had/each poem could be fitted in, grasped and understood in the moments between the medications and rounds of hospital busyness/I was learning, again, to read and write, this time in distilled foreshortened batches/I overheard hospital conversations in passing haiku-like snatches/Nothing and everything was to do with me and all was in passing/fleeting moments/

THIS BOOK IS WRITTEN AS A 'LAYERED ACCOUNT' (RONAI, 1995) IT IS ALSO A POETICS OF MEMORY, SPACE AND PLACE. It is written in the form of interlocking prose poetry, shards or shreds of 'story', verse, and fragments of academic text. These connected overlapping layers/ all catching attention in passing/ were how my life presented itself to me / under the surface was a common reprise/an interlinking musicality that was etched into the structure of time and space/ floating nearer the surface life was chaotic and disorderly/ my watch was stolen in accident and emergency when I was rushed into hospital and I found I could not make any sense of the clock on the wall/ it seemed to be going backwards/time stood still for days and then suddenly lurched forward into the following week/one moment I was getting up in the morning and in the next afternoon visiting time was over/ to quote Transtroemer again:

when a person goes so deep into a sickness that his days all
become some flickering sparks, a swarm,
feeble and cold on the horizon
(Transtroemer, *Track*, 1997)

BUT HOW WOULD/WHY SHOULD I TRANSLATE THIS JUXTAPOSITION of narrative sound/layers into written form? Once again I turned to poets whose experimentation with text and language has always lingered around the edges of our experience. From Ann Carson (1992, p. 1), whose 'glass essay' on 'hearing of little clicks inside her dream' spoke to my ways of listening to the park, I stole her form of varying the justifying borders of the text to denote different shards or fragments of story (Carson, 2003) and from myriad others from Plath to Duffy, I stole a way of ending, yet blending, sentences the one with the other by finishing not with a fullstop, but with a /. Some layers of this book are written in academic prose, others in blank verse, yet others as haiku, and all have different justifications and textual borders and fonts in the layout – a publisher's nightmare, but an author's dream/A dream with clicks and cracks inside it/ These layers are not set down on clay tablets or papyrus parchments, but on a computer that randomly and wilfully calls them /docx or jpeg40 or JStxt/...

Later I read, and layered into my account, 'at the source' by the Welsh laureate, Gillian Clarke, in her account of her writer's year/she wrote: 'It must be a memory made of layers of experience, story, snapshot, hearsay and imagination, images laid down one on the other like sedimentary rock' (Clarke, 2008, p. 51) in describing the layers that formed her poetry/this book too is formed in layers like sedimentary rock, though I would make no claims for the sparkling distillations of energy and language that make up Clarke's poetry. In this book layers and gaps between layers are left raw and unravelling before our eyes...still that mixture and messiness of inner and outer landscape, and of looking and reading is the source of this work too...

MY ETHNOGRAPHIC STUDY OF ST. ANDREWS PARK WAS INITIALLY INSPIRED BY JAY RUBY (2000) the North American anthropologist who retired from his professorship in a University in Philadelphia, back to his home town of Oak Park, Chicago, and conducted a detailed ethnography of his surroundings, spurred on by the changes that had taken place since his departure some 40 years previously. As I found myself, retired early from Bristol University on ill health grounds, sitting up in my bedroom with its large Victorian bay window overlooking the park, staring out at the life and lives entangling and unfolding before me, the ethnography began to write itself in my mind's eye.

> Today Sheila came to visit me carrying DVDs – the 'Visitor' (McCarthy, 2009) a film I had not seen – it was complex and well made/ in hospital she had sent me Tomalin's (2012) biography of Charles Dickens – a great tome – impossible for a one-handed woman to read – I could neither hold it /nor turn the pages/ the person in her mind's eye when she sent this book did not exist any longer/except in the memories of the people who had not again met me yet/if such a person existed in my memory and theirs did she/would I/ still exist?/ (I have since read the Tomalin book on my iPad/good choice)/

The stories of my relationship with my newly broken body and with the diseased horse chestnut tree opposite my window in the park, unravelled together, after my stroke, aided and abetted by my new-found practices of staring and being stared at. Thus a threefold inquiry was born out of my reciprocal relationship and entanglement with the park: my daily practices of walking in, drawing, writing about, imagining myself into and staring at the park began to form themselves into some semblance of a research method whilst a murder mystery/ ethnography/ life story/image collection also began to unfold/tangled up in the daily happenings in and of the park, and gradually leaking and spilling over/folding in on itself/ characters from the murder mystery kept crossing over into the ethnographic tales/ splinters from my own life writing broke off into other strands of the text/ there was a blurring of boundaries between different styles and images, different realisms (magical, agential and critical) and different constructions of space and time/*'Magical realism' the 'transgressive and subversive' fictional genre, whereby the magical, the mythical and the 'impossible' blend seamlessly and unapologetically with 'the actual and the real'* (Bowers, 2004)/

The writing above, in the style of Ruby, and anthropology in general, constitutes a seamless and shameless use of magical realism, in that it is written both as I have suggested, on my iPad in the bedroom bay window and also in the backroom, later in the day, in a series of versions, each gradually and cumulatively changing. Thus fieldnotes are tampered and played with. This text is no longer gleaned from participant observation, claiming Clough's ethic of 'being there' (2002, pp. 11–19). This book becomes a work of fiction, worked on at the back of the house and this working on and with the field-notes, this translation and transposition, finds these field notes doing different work. Here I make them up and exoticise them (White, 2004), they work differently here, they are no longer notes, but rather, are written up or down in academic prose and there are differences of time, place, space, aspect and, crucially, proximity to the park. In writing this I stare not at the park, but at the computer screen. I cannot see the park from the back room here. The park I am staring at in this moment is an image in my mind's eye. This is the lens through which the notes from the park, the hospital and elsewhere have been translated, or, to borrow from Eco (2004, p. 5), negotiated, into a book, since to quote, again, from Eco 'only by being literally unfaithful can a translator succeed in being truly faithful to the source text'. Indeed, Eco discovered his novels could be improved when re-embodied in a different language (p. 6). Perhaps my ethnography is improved, for it is certainly altered and displaced, by being 'literally unfaithful' to its own professed methodology?

THIS BOOK INCLUDES IMAGES AND ELEMENTS OF VARIOUS GENRES: FAIRY TALE, CRIME WRITING, SCIENCE FICTION, ETHNOGRAPHY, AUTO-ETHNOGRAPHY AND LIFEWRITING – all emerging out of my relationship and sense of inquiry into and with the place in which I live and my compulsion to draw from I saw imagined and dreamt happening outside my bedroom window/ I was and am filled with a new and renewed sense of 'dwelling place'.

The places in which
we have experienced
daydreaming
reconstitute themselves
in a new daydream,
and it is because our
memories of former
dwelling-places are
re-lived as day-dreams
that these dwelling
places of the past
remain in us for all time.

(Bachelard, 1994,
p. xxxix)

IT ALL STARTED WITH AN i-PAD. I came out of hospital just as David Hockney's one-man show at the Royal Academy came to an end, coinciding with a television documentary about his i-pad paintings of east Yorkshire landscapes (see: Hockney, 2012). As a one-handed woman who was not one of the world's 'greatest living artists' I could see that my art-making abilities were going to be more limited, but I was determined to get myself an i-pad and teach myself to use the 'brushes' app/ I often sat staring out of my bedroom window at the park, with my i-pad on my lap/this became my daily practice. Sometimes I had the 'pages' app open and sometimes I had the "brushes' app open, but writing or drawing/the i-pad was my constant companion on this project. The park was 'other' than I was. The horse chestnut was other than I was. This 'othering' led precariously to staring since 'Staring is a way of strongly reacting to another; it bespeaks involvement. It is the human response to novelty, to the unexpected' (Garland-Thompson, 2005, p. 1).

THAT NIGHT SCOSSI, MARTHA AND ABBI TRACED THE TRAIL OF FEATHERS BACK TO the house on Leopold road. The house where Scossi claimed she had seen the winged figure launch itself from the upstairs bedroom window sill. The house had three occupants, an old professor from the University, a former colleague of Abbi's, her female companion and a large blonde dog. The next morning Scossi rang the doorbell, much to the consternation of the other two. After much barking and a longish wait the professor came to the door. Scossi subjected her to quite an interrogation about the trail of turquoise feathers, which the professor did her best to answer with good grace, before shutting the door in the faces of her three neighbours.

"Christ I hope she didn't recognise me, what are you playing at, Scoss?" Said Abbi as soon as the door closed.

"I dunno ducks". Replied Scossi, "But did you notice anything odd about the way she held her shoulders?"

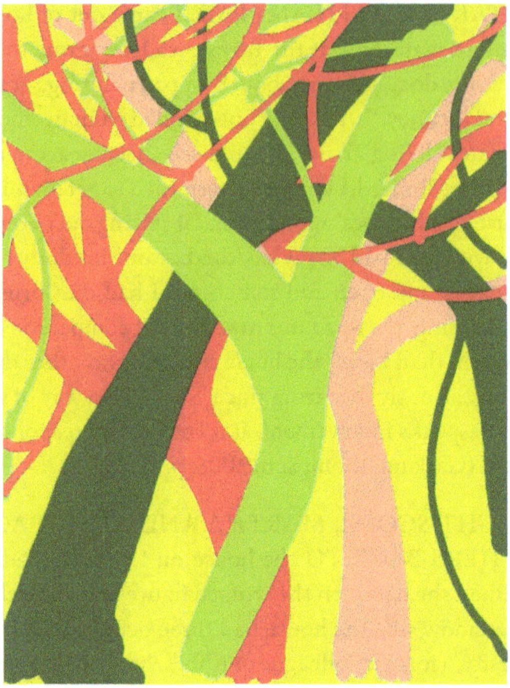

spring trees

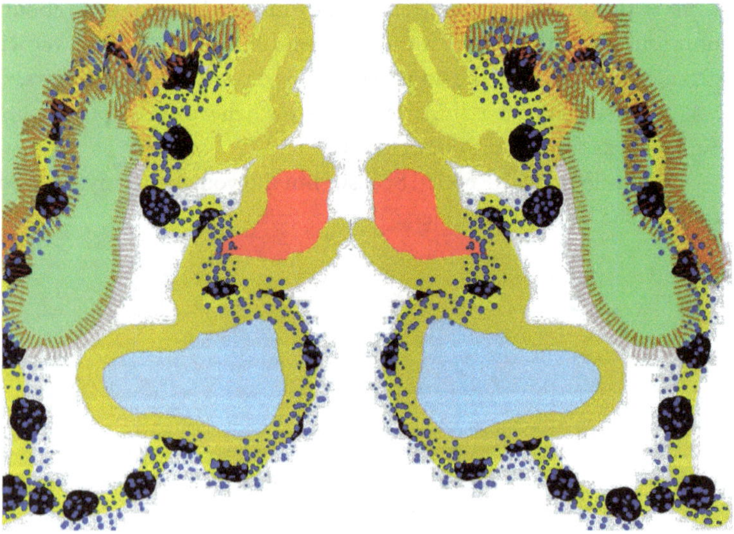

trees in conversation

WHEN I STARTED THIS STUDY, WHATEVER HAPPENED LATER, ALL THE INTERLOCKING NARRATIVES THAT MADE UP THIS BOOK BEGAN AT THEIR 'BEGINNINGS'. There was no borrowing from Woolf's beginning in the middle of life's slip stream, with a: 'Mrs Dalloway decided to buy the flowers herself' (Woolf, 1925) sentence as an opening gambit, although not only time, but linearity and chronology were problematised / played as the book progressed and, as in life, we began at first to catch glimpses of the stitching between the seams and thence to slip through some of the gaping holes we came across/then after I had abandoned the idea of three competing, contributing and interconnecting narratives, as this was not remotely my considerably more disjointed take on things; even when translated into an easier and more linear read. I was determined that this book should not be written in what James (1890) would have described as a 'stream of consciousness', a trope that others have mistranslated into 'inner monologue': both terms that seem to have been used carte-blanche for a range of twentieth/twenty-first century modernist and post-modernist novels, including Woolf (above), Joyce (1922), Plath (1963), Rushdie (1980), and Eggers (2000).

This book does contain diarised excerpts from this inner stream, such as the post card above, beginning 'today Sheila came to visit me' /this book is not an attempt to represent the inner workings, thought streams and narratives of my mind, but rather my imagined/dreamt and everyday narratives as I stared at the park/ this work does not attempt to articulate the borders or between my imagined and actual or inner and outer worlds, but rather to contest those borders/ a contestation brought into sharp focus and juxtaposition via the enormity and immense cognitive and narrative disruption of a massive stroke/ this book is the result of planting an old narrative inquirer such as myself (see Speedy, 2008) in a particular space for a very, very long time and asking her to keep her eyes, ears and what Jean Clandinin would call 'the spirit of narrative inquiry' open. This book – a poetics of a very particular emotional, geographical, storied and embodied space, the relationship between my mind and the park outside – is, in part, a response to Doreen Massey's (2000) oft-quoted claim that any space constitutes (and is constituted by) the 'simultaneity of stories thus far' that it shapes, produces and evokes/I am writing into the very particular and familiar space of the park opposite my house and engaging with, and interrogating what Clandinin and Connelly have described as the three dimensions of narrative inquiry: *people* in *contexts* over *time*. This work borrows extensively from literary and arts-based conceptualisations of these three dimensions, with the explicit intention of extending the social research imaginary. My interlocking lines of inquiry into the life of and lives lived in and around the Park weave their way through the book, disrupting and leaking into each other's style, form and content. Thus the critical realism and chronological use of time employed in the ethnographic park stories (borrowed heavily from Jay Ruby's Oak Park project), leaks and is leaked into by the magical realism and futuristic use of time from the murder mysteries. The mutual meeting space and place of the park is inscribed with the auto-ethnographic lines and disparate thoughts of my life and illness narrative/the agential realism (Barad, 2003) of the horse chestnut tree opposite my bedroom window becomes the central character at different times in different lines of flight and story, which, to borrow from Mansfield Park (Austen, 1814),'could have turned out differently, but didn't'. These three arbitrary lines of inquiry into the park – the stroke survivor's story; the murder mystery and the ethnographic study started as three texts that multiplied – defracted and became conjoint and more complex as this work progressed/ they became threads picked out of a complex interweaving that left many other stories, shards and fragments and histories hanging...

In his study of the holloways of Britain, Robert MacFarlane cites Edward Thomas (the Welsh poet) as someone who understood himself in topographical terms and believed that 'paths ran through people as sure as they ran through places' (Macfarlane, 2012, p. 20) and having sat, getting lost in a fog of my own fatigue, staring at the park for the past year(s) I now understand this certainly to be the case, though I have long imagined it to be true, that stretches of a path might carry memories of a person, just as a person might of a path. I now understand my days spent staring at the park as much in terms of a 'mapping of spectral traces' (Till, 2010) and written and drawn as much in the language(s) of cartography as of ethnography and auto-ethnography. The park runs through my being every bit as much as I long, sitting here in my wheelchair, to run through the park.

It is quite easy to lose my grip on all this intercalated storytelling: As Kurt Lindemann (2013) says

> *I lose the jagged rhizome of emotions linking disparate thoughts together like a rusty chain buried in hard-packed earth. The process of unearthing this chain does not always occur in a linear progression.*

This book, after Deleuze and Guattari (1987), is divided into plateaux and each plateau contains a variety of written shards or 'fragments'. (Plateau, according to the oxford English dictionary online, is an area of flat land higher than sea level or a period of time in which nothing changes, but the plateaux in my book are still damp from their rise above the sea and in some of them everything changes, or at least, is full of surprises like six-headed serpents rising from the depths and large winged creatures gliding in the skies above the park) This structure gives the reader something of my own experience of existing above sea level and of remembering and forgetting over the past two years and of events and meetings and persons looming up suddenly out of the fog of fatigue and, despite my extensive use of diaries – both manual and digital – the ways in which my scrambled and disjointed lack of hindsight makes for a disjointed mass of stories that conglomerate just at the entrance to my ways of organising myself and mock all forms of coherence and linearity. I had lost hold of the thread or conceit of rational, chronological narrative certainty that we all so desperately cling on to. I suspect that this ordinary, everyday way of organising our times and stories into chronologies is more of a social and temporal convenience than a reality. I always knew theoretically, that what Mark Freeman (1998) would describe as 'clock time' was a trick of the mind/light and an arbitrary human convention, but now 'what happened' has reorganised itself and continues to do so and to shift shape on a daily basis/ the journey through this book is a process of unearthing/losing a grip on the rusty chain. This old chain that links the peacock feathers on the kantha shawl (plateau 4) to the wings grown by the professor of poetic inquiry (plateau 3) is not always linear, or even linear at all, but slips beneath surfaces, unearthing itself in unlikely places. As such the elements in this work are not written as long, linear narratives, but rather as the series of short poetic interludes and prose episodes that I experienced. This is not to reify my experience as in the 'holy transcripts' (Riessman, 2008) of my research method, but in order to counter the notion of coherent chronological narrative that my experience, and I suspect, the experience of myriad others, belies. Suffering a severe stroke seriously brings into question our relationships with memory, history, clocks and time, or even 'situatedness', or at least it has for me/but perhaps we could all diverge a little from our devotion to 'clock time' in advanced western societies and bring our relationships with narrative, autobiographical, historical, environmental and mythical time a little more into focus?

AND SO IT CAME TO PASS THAT SHE ENTERED A PERIOD OF HER LIFE WHEN SHE BEGAN TO VISIT THE INFIRMARY A LOT FOR SCANS AND TAKE A LOT OF PHARMACEUTICALS (specifically bicoprolol, ramipril, warfarin and synvastatin) / They took a lot of pictures of both her brain and heart, and filed them away/ They had a kind of template and they knew what they were looking for/or so they said/Meanwhile she tended her gardens and took her medications and visited her friends and looked at her view of the park and felt the judgements of the world less harshly than she perhaps had before/ there was some comfort in this/ these things had started with a virus in the heart that had formed a blood clot that had zoomed up into her brain / it was not congenital or to do with lifestyle they said/ although she could not help wondering about the stress she had been under/they talked – the experts – both psychos and physios – about the plasticity of the brain and its relationship with memory and learning and the re-learning of old skills like walking and scratching your head/ both of which had been part of her automatic responses and had now been relegated to her forgettory/ this was all very interesting and really quite beautiful when seen in Technicolor/but there was no mention of plasticity in relation to her damaged heart/ could it regenerate?/ apparently it could/ apparently it has/she is pronounced, some two years later/ once again a woman of good heart

> What she really wanted to know was where her immense imaginarium was located and/or if her imaginarium was located at all or was unfixed and just floating about/they spoke knowledgeably about the damaged right side of her brain which controlled the weakened left side of her body and of her prefrontal cortex which regulated emotion and was undamaged (but what about the inappropriate laughter?) and of her equally intact amygdala, which connected what was happening in the world to her emotions/ but this was not her pressing concern/ Indeed she had often thought as she got older that she had/out of necessity and the desire to survive/ had a rather overactive prefrontal cortex as a child and if a little less regulation around emotion was on the agenda/ well, bring it on/what she really wanted to know was – where was the bit of her brain that had always been so good at connecting what was **not** necessarily happening to her thoughts and feelings/aka her imaginarium/for she was blessed with an

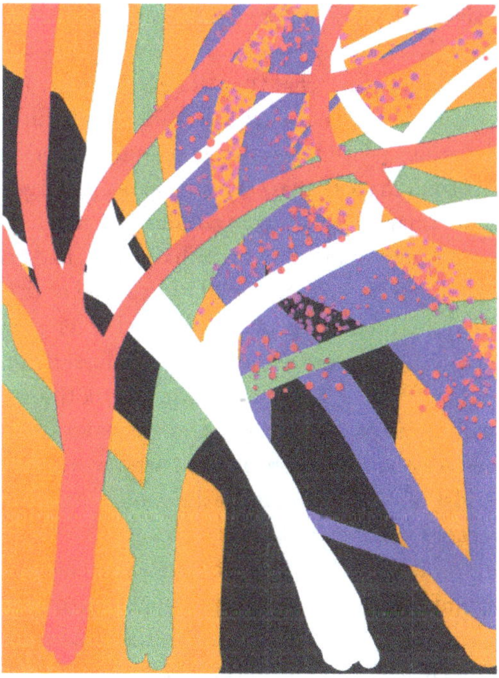

summer trees

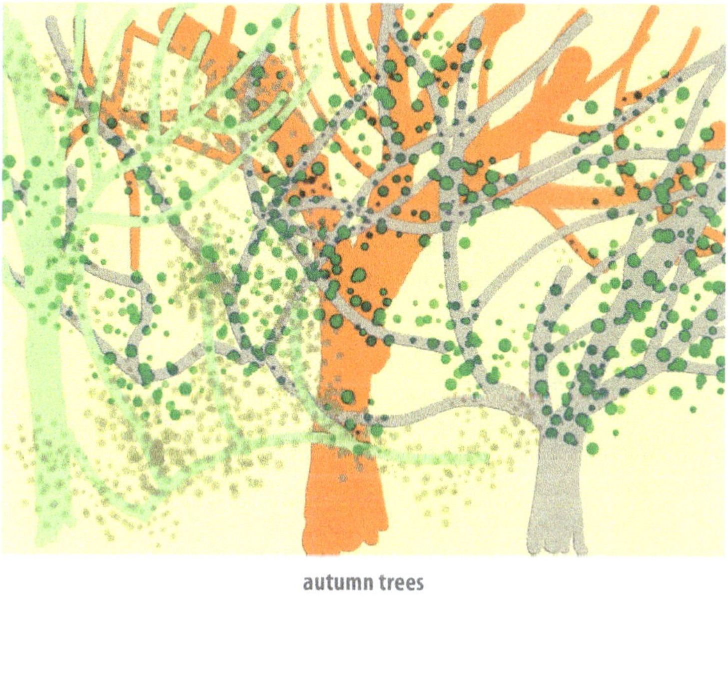

autumn trees

extensive perceptive and preternaturally predictive imaginarium that had always compelled her to see what they did not wish her to see and to notice what they did not wish her to notice and to hear what they did not wish her to hear/ she did not carry this facility around with her just for the human world but for plants too and trees in particular/ she did not necessarily feel distraught about her imaginarium waning/indeed for much of her life being able to imagine so much in such sharp relief had been quite hard work/it might be quite peaceful to let some of this go/ it would just be quite interesting to know if and when she was going to imagine less/ she perhaps just wanted to gently imagine herself into a space where her imagination was not quite so vivid and compelling/a life less imagined might have a serenity about it and serenity had always been her friend when she had found it/ It was just that for the moment she couldn't quite imagine it/and nobody else seemed bothered/

there was much talk of memory and identity/even memory narrative and identity/ she was clear that remembering and imagining were not the same/memory often had to do with the way things were and a bit less of that might be a bit of a tonic in life/ she was quite engaged for the moment with the way things might yet become and couldn't quite see her way out of that engagement any day soon but/she was not sure exactly what percentage of her current identity was to do with remembering (particularly as she had put some considerable effort into forgetting over the years) and how much was to do with imagining or indeed quite what the signal to noise ratio between remembering imagining and forgetting actually was/she knew she had some memory problems (although she had not yet placed her purse in the fridge and the portobellini mushrooms in her handbag – that would be just silly)/ she was not having any trouble imagining all kinds of stuff and seemed very capable of forgetting quite a lot/the medical literatures did not seem to worry about the imaginarium so perhaps she shouldn't either/ it's just that (and this is just between ourselves) although she very much appreciated the efforts of all these eloquent inquirers (King, 2000) to string together myriad connexions between memory, identity and narrative/ her identity had always been more fluid and tended to shift shape and leak more than these texts seemed to allow for/ she had learned over the years to sit lightly/ half listening/ to other people's stories about her/quietly making up her own and then sliding through small spaces and slippery doorways when she thought she might be caught up with/caught out/so really she knew that remembering was not all that – and identities could be lightly taken off like cardigans in summer/she would just like to know what to take for a bit of light preventative imaginarium maintenance/ she could not believe it was anything like turmeric and black pepper and she had a gently held fancy (see what I mean) that it would be something or a combination of things growing in her own garden/right under her nose/if she could just get a little whiff of it on the wind/perhaps if she went out into the park/

POSITIONED AS BOTH STARER AND STAREE in relation to the park that is being inquired into/the researcher used not only practices of listening, but also of looking/this work involved hard staring: a harsh, interlocking engagement and visual entanglement with the park, as well as a kind of reverie or soft semi-inward gazing/it includes both landscapes and dreamscapes real and imagined and evokes the production of deduced, induced and imagined knowledges/ borders between fact and fiction were interrogated and thresholds between different forms of realism: agential, critical and/or magical/were breached/

Last night I dreamt that I was running across the park/The quickest way across to the Gloucester road/where I was headed/is to run straight down the hill across the grass/in my dream I ran down the winding tarmac path towards the Effingham road entrance/I was in bare feet/ wearing my green cotton nightie

Running through Bristol/an old estuary port city/captured by the stench and darkness/ hostage to stone tapes/keepers of centuries of intrigue, bloodshed and violent outbursts with dagger and spray can down dark alleyways/I run on in careless anticipation/ Pissnfishhead passageways opening onto silent squares where lonely trees eke out their celibate city lives/leaning into triangular trade winds in the vain hope of airborne fruitfulness/disjuncture and entanglement/

DISJUNCTURE AND ENTANGLEMENT/I was hospitalised for three months/I spent my mornings for the next two years at home/ mostly sitting in an upright armchair/sometimes wheelchair in my bedroom/ staring out of the bay window at the park opposite/**this book is written in the way things happened**/ according to Sameshima (2007, p. 286) 'the use of an alternate format can significantly open new spaces for inquiry'/ large swathes of fogginess were cut across – breached even – by great humpbacked mounds of clarity/ have I told you all this before?/very possibly/this book is a sea shanty from a landlubber adrift on her own in a seaport fog/I have been dreaming that my body was a text / an old mouldy leatherbound book/ left out in the damp of the park/ there the dark hole in my head which must have previously contained some very useful information like how to raise the middle finger of my left hand and point it at the sky in disdain and disbelief/life has seemed both disjointed and entangled and so is this sea of stories/the disjuncture comes from this drifting/this being all at sea in a familiar life/and yet I am not alone in this fog /there are all sorts of other people and things bobbing about /bumping up against them in a haphazard disjointed kind of way has led to all kinds of entanglements/caught in nets and networks/I find myself entangled in constellations of objects and people that I did not see coming /suddenly thrown up along with broken shells and bits of dried up weed on unknown shores/the hole in my head was filled with wet sand that had got in through the crevices in my skull/it was that pure/white bay-of-islands kind of sand/full of golden sea slug creatures wriggling in and out of my skull/in the park, I found a woman in the hedge/

]

]

]

[

[

[ ]

]

this was not the kind of hedge you got close to/it was not until you came across it that you knew where you were/even then she could not – hand on heart – say she'd reached it/she just slipped through into the cobwebbed thickets where she could still pick out shapes, hear far-off voices and glimpse shadows in the mirrors as she passed/ only then – if she made it – might she look back for a split-second towards the surface of that other hedge/next thing you notice?/she'd be gone/

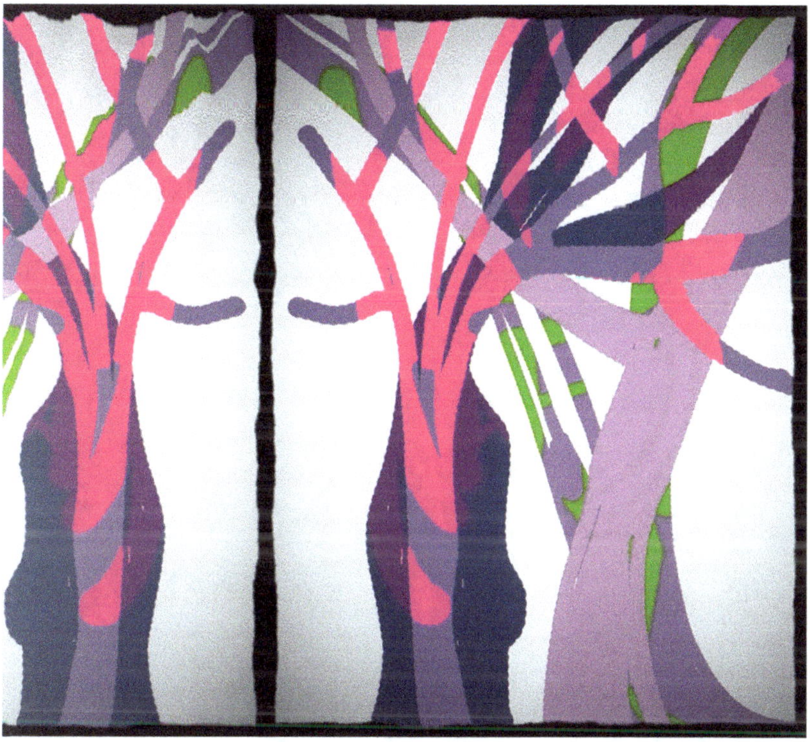

more trees in conversation

Second plateau

A process of writing developed eventually or at least a method of/pdf

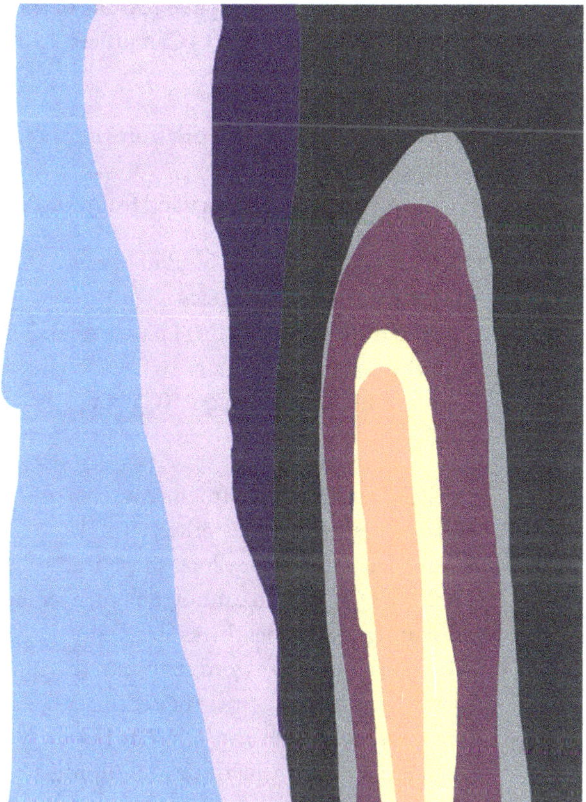

spring in the park

Starring at the Park: A Poetic Autoethnographic Inquiry, Jane Speedy, 45–92.

OR AT LEAST A METHOD OF PLACING ALL THE SCRAPS TOGETHER; alongside, in juxtaposition, emerged/staring then writing or drawing/staring again/blatant scrutiny of a local habitation with a name/ St. Andrews Park/chronicled/staring collected the scraps for the book, images retained in the drawing: an 'ars memoria' of the mind: 'monastic memoria is more like what is called now "mindfulness" than what many psychologists deem to be memory, a discipline of attentive recollection and concentrated reading of texts in the bible (lectio divina)' (Carruthers, 2008, p. 154).

Scraps and fragments of work from Sappho,
written on papyrus,
float in on the red dust of a wind from Africa:

'they arrived. But you, O blessed one,
smiled in your deathless face
and asked what (now again) I have suffered
and why
(now again) I am calling out' (Carson, 2003, p. 3)

I write these scraps and fragments from my life
and toss them to the westerlies,
In imitation of a heroine long since dead,
unlike her Gods, who cannot, do not, ever die,
presenting us with deathless faces,
We grasp at Sappho's words between the
silences and blanks across the centuries/
I imagine into her spaces/I imitate these
scratchings with my justifications/borders/
edges/
verges that draw lines down and across my
scribbled notes from times in hospital/etched
onto the scraps where I start to write my

musings on the park/she has papyrus that we
will yet find/I have an iPad that justifies the
edges of my text/

> My own writing bullies me
> Into attempting a back somersault
> Lands me on my back
> It looks dynamic, flying through the air
> But you've got to score the landing

AND SOME OF YOU ARE CONCERNED
With how my words sit on the page
This work in stanza form/squeezed into the centre of the page/
You try to work out reasons for these line breaks which some
times chop WO
RDS in half/
Funnelled down the page/
Is this intentional or just a formatting error, you ask?

OLD BITS OF CLOTH, LEFT ON AN ISLAND BY SAPPHO/ 'Breaks are always' to quote Derrida (1981, p. 24) , 'and fatally, re-inscribed in an old cloth that must continually and interminably, be undone'
Translators, like Anne Carson (2003, p. xi) use square brackets 'to give an impression of missing matter' or 'the presence of letters not quite legible'.... Not every gap or space or illegibility is indicated as 'this would render the page a blizzard of marks and would inhibit reading' similarly I leave an uneasy silence when you ask for justifications of all my margins, verges and justifications as this would render the text awash with justifications for my formatting/narrow margins are probably just that/equally wide verges/The gaps are where the excitement lies for the reader who sees them as part of the text/it is a visual text/ and all about staring into space and walking down narrow passages/ 'brackets imply a free space of imaginal adventure' (p. xi):

And we are left, from Sappho, the lyricist, with:

']
  ]
  ]
  ]thought
  ]barefoot
  ]
  ]
  ]'

(Carson, 2005, p. 12)

and our imaginings/in the spaces/where the writing has faded/

and I am left/
staring at the park/marked and spattered with
spectral traces/mapped by foxes and humans
along pathways/
stories of the park and recent memories
of the hospital /an absent presence both in life and in the NHS/
that seems larger and more substantive and densely peopled than
the rest of life/ standing alone without a
blizzard of
justifications/frail/

THE NOTES FROM MY DAYS IN THE HOSPITAL TWO YEARS AGO /PRESERVED IN TWO NOTEBOOKS/ are faded in places and water-stained/I too use square brackets in my text to 'give an impression of missing matter' ... not lost over centuries/but over circumstances/

the fragments we have from the texts of the ancients were recorded by scribes onto papyrus sheets and written down in straight, narrow columns – as if taken from oral renditions / giving no hint of spacing or intonation
(Carson, 2003, pp. ix–xiii) I have tried to emulate this style in my own text/writing in narrow columns as if listening and translating my thoughts and imaginings whilst staring at the park/ taking them down in translation/ the stanzas and spacing indicating not the rhythms the author envisaged in the flow of

the work, but the gaps and disjunctures between fragments of thoughts/stories/found poems in conversations overheard/

BORROWED

FORMS FROM
ANCIENT POETS/ORAL WORKS
INSCRIBED WITH TWENTY-FIRST CENTURY
TECHNOLOGIES/ marks made on paper in narrow
columns/ emulating ink

The earliest writing was found on clay tablets...
contemporary stains and
emulations made by

forma
tting
proce
sses
and
drop-
down menu
s
/choi
ces to justify selected

> this compels you to wonder about what writing is, how it came about more than five thousand years ago and what the world might have looked like without it
>
> (Finkel, 2014, p. 262)

> all cuneiform signs had more than one sound value and all sounds could be represented by more than one cuneiform sign, or in other words, polyvalence is all
>
> (Finkel, 2014, p. 425)

work/whole documents or
lonely only paragraphs/
the poetic inquirers, both
linguistic and literary (see
Prendergast, Leggo and
Sameshima, 2009) tell us
that verse in stanza is the

closest written form to
spoken words/ but I invite
the readers to construct their
own stanzas and accents
from my narrow columns/
translated from snatches of
conversation buried in some
pocket of my mind/

like discarded tissues in
cardigansleeves/these scraps
are slowly teased out/

STARING AT THE
PARK/ IPAD IN
HAND/ SOMETIMES
DRAWING/SOMETIMES
WRITING/a bag of books
nearby/ another load on
hand online/ along with
online readings/poetry/
stories/ academic papers/
Carol Rambo Ronai and
her layers meets Carol Ann
Duffy and her gospels/
Gillian Clarke and her
poetics
from the source (where
'other ghosts have left their
traces and their names/
Some are benign ghosts
whose lost habitations are
marked only by the nettles
and gooseberry bushes
that show they were ever
there' [2011, p. 4]) meets
Stephanie Springgay and her
allies (2005) in a/r/tography
which claims, borrowing

from Maxine Greene
(1995) that 'the arts have
the distinct power to open
our imagination toward
the unimagined and the
uncertain' / this will
become a many-layered, sed-
imentary book/

FULL STOPS SEEM
SOMEHOW TOO FULL/
JUST DIAGONAL LINES
SEEM MORE appropri-
ate/borrowed from Anne
Carson and her red stories[1]/
edges and borders to spill
over rather than stops in the
writing/
And then the outside creeps
inside/inside the room and
inside the woman/And
Susanne finds in the slants/
Shades of Emily Dickinson
who urged us to tell: 'all the
truth but tell it slant'[2]/ This
slanted text tells what I see/
tells all the truths that hard
core staring can dig out of
a life/park/mind/in the fog
between us

RUSTLING IN THE
CORNER/ COMING
IN THROUGH THE
WINDOW/that opens onto
the park/blurring the edges
between outside and inside
the house/between outside
and inside my mind/maybe

a squirrel or a fox? Perhaps a
bird or another, more exotic
form of winged creature/
has become trapped behind
the dressing table?/
perhaps there is a badger,
escaping the cull, hiding
in the bedroom alcoves,
behind the wardrobe?/

I SIT THERE IN THE
WINDOW and my mind
wanders back to a conversation
with Mabel, my neighbour on
the stroke ward/Perhaps I am
losing my marbles?
'If you cry they'll
offer you
anti-
depressants'/'but I
have
a lot to cry about/
yesterday
I cried because I
could not
get my own knickers
on/
that's all'/and then
came
the ward round/ in
hierarchical order
/the consultant
suggests
antidepressants /
again/
stroke patients get
depressed
/it seems/and little

pills transform their
lives /I'm told
/'but I have a lot to
cry about'/ I argue /
'well I cannot force
you'/
she smiles/tight-
lipped /like a nun
faced with a sinner/
which is the greatest
sin? The crying or the
pill refusal? / Forgive
me father for I did
not take my pills/ I
took the
anticoagulants and
the beta blockers/
but not the cytalo-
pram/ I am familiar
with the side
effects/ and
do not want
them/what's
more I do not
think they
should be
handed
out to all these
old ladies with
vascular
dementia like
sweeties/ what
is going
on here ? /why
shouldn't the
elderly
and infirm be
allowed to cry?

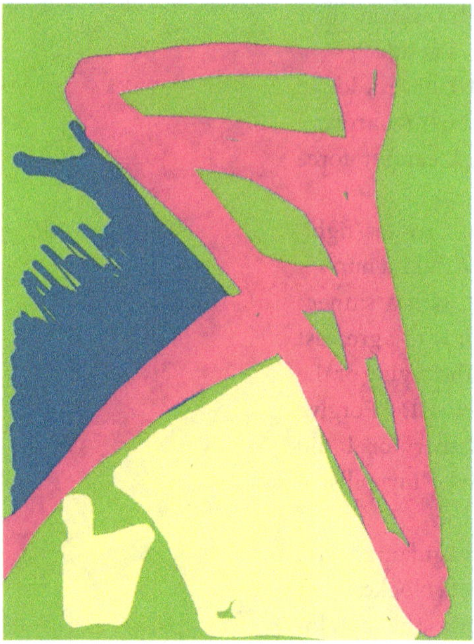

summer in the park

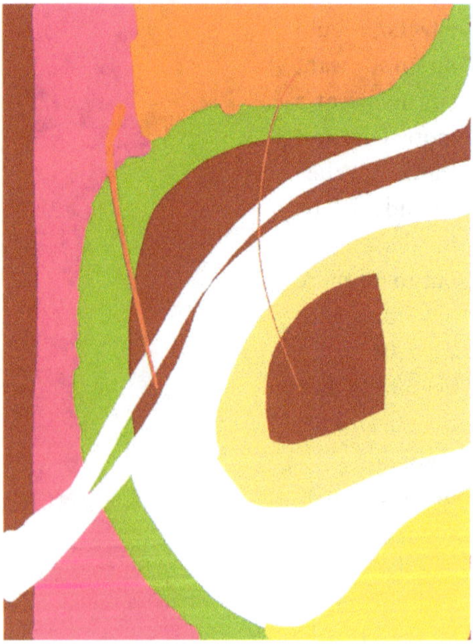

autumn in the park

/There
is a lot to cry
about/ why not
let us all
sit and cry/and
cry and cry/
Where is
the harm in
that?/Who are
these pills for
the patients or
the staff?/It is
difficult
for the staff/ I
am told/ if you
are all in
tears all the
time/but it was
just this once/ and
once again before
Christmas/and when
you first came
here/ OMG is
there a 'how
many times
she cried' chart
as well as a
'Bristol
stools chart'
in that folder?
/ Did Robert
McCrum cry?
Does Andrew
Marr? / are
they taking
cytalopram?/
What about
those North

Americans who
talked to Oprah
about their
strokes of
insight? /or
are they too
'enlightened'
for anti-
depressants?

MEMORIES THE PARK
KEEPS SAFE/memories I
keep safe in the park
all our landscapes are
littered with memories/
leaves/other traces/and are
open to our dreams/

an award-winning green
space/
criss-crossed with
tarmacadammed paths/dog
tracks/fox-runs/thoughts/
ideas/imaginings/layers
of dust/leaves and things
we just forgot/someone
traverses the park in a
wheelchair/
at first I think it is Sue
coming here/but why would
she be coming in a chair/
when she can come in her
car?/ And I remember the
time that she lent us her
cottage in Laugharne/...

I WAS SITTING ON THE
SOFT LEATHER SOFA
not wanting to leave/What's

> The huge repository of the memory, with its secret and unimaginable caverns, welcomes and keeps all these things, to be recalled and brought out for use when needed.
>
> (Carruthers, 2008, p. 139)

to leave for now that we have
rigged up a system for the
dog not trying to commit hari
kiri down the bank every
five seconds?/we have all
the windows open and the
warm sun is streaming in on
our faces/It is mid-October,
but I have a slight tan from
yesterday's walk/Sarah
is reading/I am writing a
paper/or was/I am currently
writing this/tomorrow I have
meetings all day/and here we
are, a couple of hours from
home, watching cormorants
arch their wingpits (is this
cormorant for 'come and
get me'?) and listening to
the lament of the curlews/
down below us, a man with a
basket is gathering something
(samphire?) from the water's
edge as the tide goes swiftly
out/ yesterday we met a local,
Bob, on the cliff path who
remembered Dylan Thomas
from when he (Bob) was a boy.

Whilst we were chatting I/
being a bit of a show off (surely
not)/had recited/falteringly/
the first words of under milk
wood:

'It is spring, moonless
night in the small town,
starless and bible-
black, the cobble streets
silent.....'

Whereupon Bob had
launched into an impeccable
rendition of the whole two and
a half pages of the first speech
of 'first voice' in a beautiful,
lilting local baritone/He does
this regularly in the town
hall by all accounts, but was
very courteous about my very
'English' attempt at the first
few words .../

Interesting place this..../

We will pack up shortly and
trundle off home/Bummer/

NAPOLEON
BONAPARTE KNEW
THAT AN ARMY
MARCHES ON IT'S
STOMACH, JUST AS I
KNOW THAT ***I WRITE***
FROM MY STOMACH.
Unlike Napoleon's army,
my writing has nothing to

do with what, or how much
I eat, indeed, if my writing
is flowing well I often
forget to eat at all/I have a
particular 'on edge' tummy
feeling when my writing
is going well/when I am
in what Csikszentmihalyi
(2002) would describe as
'flow' in writing, this feeling
comes from my stomach/
it is as if the writing is all
buried down there inside
and when the timing is right
the words just flow up and
float off and mingle with
the external world/it is an
embodied – (both *from*
and *in* the body) process/
it is the feeling of making
something, or of something
in the making flowing
from and *through* me/it
is a feeling of connecting
to the world, as Gauntlett
(2011) says 'making is
connecting' and my writing
in 'flow' definitely makes
connections in the world/
writing is traditionally
viewed as a cerebral,
intellectual process, but
in my case writing is a
practice involving not only
what Weems (2003) would
describe as the imagination-
intellect but also the whole

core of my body/writing
is a practice of making
connections that I can still
engage with and feel the
same about, despite having
had a stroke 18 months ago
which has left me with a
huge amount of left-sided
weakness/paralysis/I may
be a one-handed writer these
days, but I can still achieve a
'flow' that the world around
me sustains/it is a flow
through inner and outer
bodies/ landscapes, the one
informing/connecting/
overlapping with/leaking
into the other/it is a leaky
and broken body of work/
drawing is the same, evokes
the same feelings/and
Andrew Marr (2013, p. 34)
too cites Csikszentmihalyi
and this feeling of flow in
relation to drawing:
'work which absorbs you,
mind and body, at the peak
of your concentration and
skill'

Both the iPad drawing and
writing in this work are
drawn and written as 'flow'
from my tummy/embodied/
this book progresses on its
stomach...

AMONGST THE
FRAGMENTS OF THESE
WRITTEN NARRATIVES,
THREE VISUAL narratives
unfold: finger paintings that
the trees drew out of me/
abstract images that I drew
out of the landscape/and
the emergent edges of the
visual method and limits
put on my mark-making by
the iPad/the trees in the
park evoked the first finger
paintings/I opened the iPad,
opened the 'brushes' app
and began to translate what
I saw onto the screen? /not
so much translate, as make
visible, what is possibly
there/make visible what
can be abstracted from the
scene/not representing or
reproducing, but lay down
the sedimentary testimonies
that lie beneath/alongside
and in connection with/
there is something really
satisfying about drooling
the bright clear colours out
of the ends of my fingers,
this kind of painting
evokes memories of play /
getting sticky/then came
the pictures of aerial views
of the pathways/ multiple
images of the peacock
feathered kantha shawl
rendered repeatedly in

the reflections app /the
kinds of marks the tools
could make began to
both expand and limit the
images I produced/I began
to yearn for messier mark
making and to hanker after
large sticks of charcoal,
soft, textured handmade
papers, bristly hog's hair
brushes and bottles of
thick oily Indian ink/but a
one-handed woman could
not easily carry all these
materials up to her bedroom
and clear away the debris
later/ I made a brutal,
pragmatic decision to stick
with the iPad and its clean,
digital marks/
I was restricted by my
mobility, my handedness
and my tools/ struck by both
the smallness and enormity
of my chosen project/my
experience of this corner of
the park, set down with what
I could carry in one hand to
record its stories/these were
the parameters of my study/

I WAS IN A HOSPITAL THAT WAS CLOSING DOWN/ IN A WARD BUILT WITH MONIES DONATED BY THE WORKERS OF BRISTOL/ now sold to become luxury harbour-side flats/a sea of conversation overheard/found poems from the end of the ward/I took notes/notebooks full of talk interspersed with my comments:

I can see silhouettes of people in the Redcliffe flats/ Shadowy figures stretched across the landings/ Lights in rows of three glaring down on the hospital opposite/below/this building has been sold to property developers /quality retail and luxury flats/ It looks like a workhouse, but it was built as a hospital in 1832/ a lovely Bristol stone building/a prime site/ yellow and black tape around the windows/take away the double glazing and there's a two inch gap through to the outside/those tiles on the ceiling/that's where a leak came in/

I remember coming to visit our Barry in here when he was a kid/ There was Gynae in here as well as the old ... and infirm/I had the last hysterectomy in here, she said/ just before... /

Elsie: Perhaps I'll have a little drink/ Tea/two sugars please./

MrsK; Makit. Da faucer da klausdi

Elsie: oh shut up/I can't understand a word you're saying...../

MrsK: Makit, no......

Mavis: Len brought me earplugs do you want some?

Jane: no thanks/they hurt my ears/ I'm going to listen to the radio through my headphones while they fight it out/

Mavis: Sorry, can't hear you, got me earplugs in...

Have you filled yours in? I've read it, but I haven't filled it in. I can't bear the fact that we're all going to be split up by this after all this time. What shifts are you going to do? Are you going to do 2 long days?

I can't do that it's too stressful for me/

The new linen service is ridikerlus, ridikerlous. There's no nighties/ Well make do with pyjama tops, then/

FILLING IN THE DLA FORMS*/ TODAY I AM IN A BLEAK MOOD/I HAVE BEEN FILLING IN MY FORMS FOR THE GOVERNMENT/they want to know how disabled I am/they want a list of what I cannot do/this is negative bragging/I fill in the questions about walking and about eating and about peeing and about pain/ there are no questions about laughing or friendship or poetry or painting/ only about my limitations/I see the sense in this, but it boxes me in and leaves me feeling hopeless and bleak/ I want to shout at 'them'/to have toddler tantrums/it seems such an indignity on top of so many others/I want to shout: bloody fucking Tory bastards/ that was what was wrong with Robert McCrum's memoir: he was so posh that none of the form filling stuff affected him/he had no idea how disability affects people who are not the literary editor of the Observer/I suppose as a professor I am protected too/ I have a pension as well as DLA ....*
Mary Weems speaks from the wound in her mouth, whilst I stutter from the hole in my head/what a life/ what a bunch.../

IN THE HOSPITAL, THE TALK CAME
FLOATING ROUND ME THROUGH THE FOG/
you need to apply for your own job by January 2nd/
you need to put down three choices or they may
slot you in one of theirs/well really if the NHS isn't
working I think they ought to sort out the top/ not
bands 3–6/'weeding out'/'losing people'/surely it's
the senior management that's to blame/

This man/A suit/ came to audit the stroke ward/
He was surrounded by people working/nurses talking to people/giving out medicines from trolleys/getting old ladies into their clothes/
Physios helping people move along the ward, clutching frames and sticks/but he wasn't interested/he did not look up once/he just sat
there with the files/ and read the tick sheets/
and made a note where pages or charts were missing/he did not care what they were doing/
just as long as they had recorded it correctly/

you can't get out of bed sweetheart/
you are going to fall/
you don't need to move you are fine there/
I'm still here/ I'm not going anywhere/
Just seeing if I can go to the toilet

I was, (to quote Grace Mccleen, 2013, p. 346)
'Awash on a current, a slick of debris, words, papers, scraps, shards, years dispersing itself over darkening waters'...

Black and white stripey tee shirt
Black soft woolly trousers
Black bra (top of wardrobe)
Brigid Jones style pants
Any socks/
All is vague chaotic, uncertain mess

Why am I not getting my brain into gear?

Why am I not walking down the ward by now?

HAPPY NEW YEAR/THEY ARE LOSING STAFF/
STRANGE THING TO LOSE/losing car keys but not people/ Losing has an accidental air about it/ sacking sounds deliberate/losing nurses – a nurse is quite a large item to lose/In the new hospital there will be a ward for 30 people, twice as big as this/there are fewer jobs and more patients/

Yes/They are making 2 wards into one/ so there will be less jobs/but they are appointing less trained staff/ so people like me will be doing more of the jobs now undertaken by the trained staff/more of the medical stuff/painkillers and cholesterol/here are your tablets/happy new year/

ELSIE IS GROANING RHYTHMICALLY FROM AN OPEN MOUTH/no-one should die alone/ Elsie has been dying ever since she came in/She is dying here with us/ not her loved ones/ not her chosen ones/
I feel it is her choice to be in here/knowing nothing of her wishes/there was a niece who came once/had a conference with the consultant about the care plan/ and then vanished/silence/so we are to be her companions at her death/our softer breathing accompanies her groans in the cool night air/ it is January 1st, 2012/ Elsie has seen in the new year/ surely she will not die tonight? /
Is she in pain? I ask/I should think so dear/how old is she? I ask/ I think about 83/Edna replies/

I WATCH HER BREATH IN OXYGEN THROUGH A MASK and take up food through her tube and I wonder about assisted death and life and death and medicine/ if she were my dog I would know what to ask them for/ this does not seem quite right to me/ not quite humane/ and yet we remain here and her silent witnesses on the ward/what do the nurses think/ I wonder/ perhaps they do not question tonight's news item on assisted death/discussed in the house of lords/a new report in the law lords (Warnock, 2012) /with Elsie in their mind's eyes/perhaps they do/and we the witnesses surround her aching body with our breath/our human presence/for we will be the mourners when she goes/an absence lingering still amidst our presence/

HUMANS ARE ANIMALS AND LIKE ALL ANIMALS WE LEAVE TRACKS AS WE WALK: signs of passage made in snow, sand, mud, grass, dew, earth or moss (Macfarlane, 2012). As we cross and criss the park going about our daily lives, we leave traces, scents and stories of our coming and our going: palimpsests that can offer readings into the architecture of our lives. It was these traces, scents and stories that she was mapping from her window: recording these inscriptions on the park and their indentations into the life of the park itself/in the snow she could see clearly the tangle of dog, fox, bird, squirrel, rat, human, bicycle and buggy tracks making their way across the park/ the foxes take possession of the landscape at night/it is only in the early morning, after it has snowed, that their journeys back and forth can be mapped by humans/many of them live in lairs buried down beneath the park keeper's huts on the corner of Effingham and Melita road, but some come into the park at night from the surrounding houses and gardens/ looking down into her own garden the morning after it had snowed, she could see fox tracks winding their way along the front path and across the road into the park. She had heard them howling and mewling in the night over on the other side of the park. The thing about the pattern

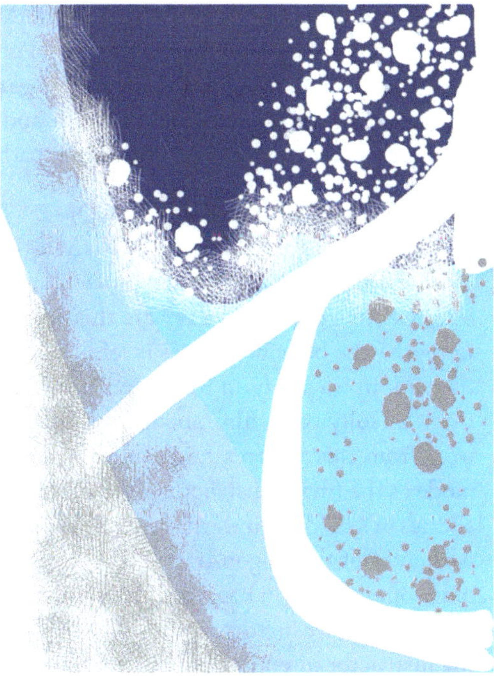

winter in the park

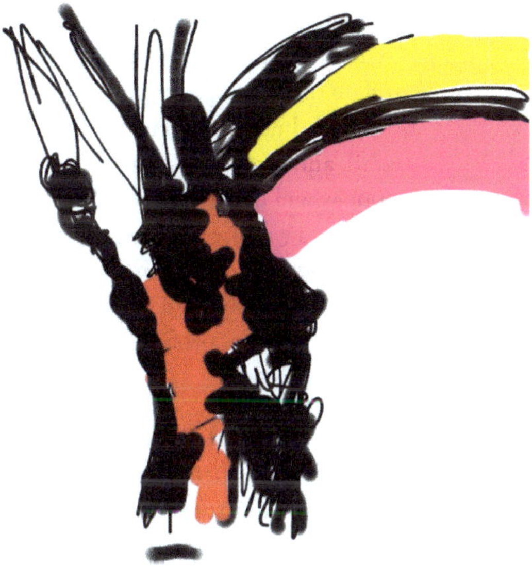

horse chestnut again

of fox tracks was that they always looked the same, it was as if the tangle of fox pathways that only ever appeared visible and subject to the human gaze when it snowed, was as inscribed into the fabric and memory of the park as the concrete and tarmac paths/

THE YUMMY MUMMIES COME THREE TIMES A WEEK IN THE SPRING, SOMETIMES MORE/they come in designer kit wielding designer buggies: lime green and navy are this year's colours for both/ the bevy of buggies is left in the centre of the park in wagon-train formation/it is like a scene from a Hollywood film about 'how the west was won'/from this we go straight into Busby Berkeley mode as the (male) instructor leads the mummies in a series of syncopated warm-up exercises around the perimeter of the wagon train, some involving skipping ropes and bean bags/gradually different posses of mummies are lured away from the buggy-train by the instructor into a series of increasingly elaborate circuits around the park's outer pathways, leaving their buggies in the centre in the care of one or two their fellow mummies/there are always one or two who are not prepared to leave their buggies who set off on these escapades pushing their progeny in front of them, but they soon give up on the overland buggy trail and even those in the range-rover-discovery four-wheel drive buggy bracket give up eventually/ there is a waiting list for these classes/how shall I put this?/ people of African-Caribbean and Asian origin are particularly underrepresented in this yummy mummy group, although, funnily enough, not in this area of Bristol/

the circus school students tended to stay inside during the snow/that week there had been no hoopla-hooping, tight-rope walking or African drumming practice in the park/perhaps the drummer was annoying his own neighbours that week as much as he had annoyed the people living around the park for the past month? Or perhaps he was finally learning a different rhythm?/ Tai-chi and drug dealing both continued despite the snow/A small group of dedicated, pyjama-clad Tai-chi do-ers gathered every morning beneath the Maurice road plane trees. They moved separately, and also somehow together, in slow motion, across the east side of the park, facing the sun rise/below them, on the drug dealing bench, it was business as usual/this morning it was the red-headed bloke with the beard who seemed to have brought endless supplies with him in the pockets of his duffle coat/'what if one of the Tai-chi doers was an under-cover cop?' she asked herself. "what if I were an undercover cop?'...... /she began to turn over newspaper headings in her mind's eye 'retired Professor of Education uncovers Bristol drugs cartel' 'Ethnographer identifies drug dealers in her local park' .....which led her onto other imagined scenarios .....'snooping professor found murdered with her own binoculars in her bedroom'...

THE HORSE CHESTNUT STANDS IN THE PARK OUTSIDE MY WINDOW/
it is about the same age as the house/ the park is Victorian too/ we moved in thirteen years ago, in the spring/the tree was just coming into leaf/ each year new leaves decorate the bell of its branches /each May its buds have burst into dark pink blossom candelabras

/ her green-tinged bark is covered in knurled wooden fungus-like lumps/ but I have never worried about them before/ only this year/ when I had the time/when I was spoilt for time/ did I stop and look closely at the tree and see the dark dank patch in the fork of her trunk/ canker/ Horse Chestnut canker/ the Oak tree behind has a kindred woody fungus/ but not the bleeding from the trunk/the horse chestnut tree is weeping shamelessly and I have never even noticed/ how many years has she stood there weeping darkly in front of my window while I have carried on with life?/

year upon year for thirteen years I have neglected the passing of the seasons in this city/ every year we plan to go to Westonbirt to catch the Autumn colours in the arboretum and find that once again we have missed the moment/
year upon year I wait until we travel in the summer to Pembrokeshire / or at

new year/ our bi-annual sojourn in the country and only then/ out of the city and away from the routines of our everyday lives/ I notice the passing of the seasons/ At new year I notice that I have once again missed the turn into Autumn/ the falling and turning of the leaves/ in the summer I perceive greenness / shooting
]

new growth/ for the rest of the year/I live here/ in the company of the park/ I live daily next to the horse chestnut, and I never notice how she is/

But this
year is
different

]
]
]
]

[ ]

]
]
]
]

[ ]

/DECEMBER 28TH/ AN INCIDENT/ A NOISE IN THE NIGHT/The oak tree next to the horse chestnut is down/ ripped at the fork of her trunk, her longest and heaviest branch has fallen into the park/ no-one is hurt/ bald-headed men come and look at the damage/ neighbourhood conversations take place/I watch different groups of people come and stand around the fallen tree/ all day people come with hacksaws and chain saws to glean pieces and branches for their fireplaces/by nightfall the fallen treetop is bare. /January 3rd/when we

come back from Wales the stripped-bare tree is lying in pieces in the park/people pass by and try and pick up the logs/ but they are too big for them to carry/ everything that can be taken home already has been/these great logs are waiting for the park keepers to clear them/my horse chestnut looks on/ still bleeding furiously from the middle/wondering

what her faithful companion has done to garner all this human attention/no-one notices her weeping/ it is getting very cold and her twigs and branches are covered in a film of frost every morning/not only am I alongside the Horse Chestnut/watching and

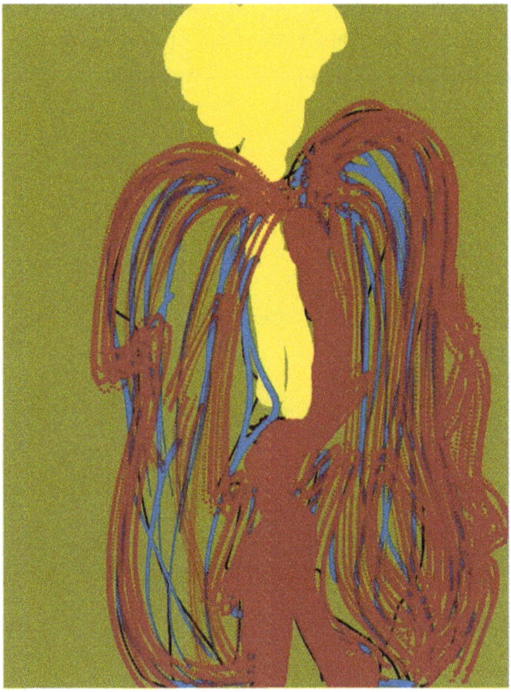

angel from mars

waiting and idling and staring/but she is

also alongside me / so vibrantly

THE ANGELS FROM MARS BLOW DOWN THEIR SMOKY BREATH TO EARTH/ THEIR BLUE VEINED WINGS/disguising golden tresses/
and intergalactic ironmongery blackened in the foundries of their ancient planet/they swoop down like rusty dragons/ creaking and groaning across our skies/the chain-bone structure of their external skeletons rustling/ in a fibrous expectant dance/whilst they choose which one of us / to take back as their prey/

We have our own stories to live by and fondly narrate our selves as something more than angel fodder From the myths of ancient Mars/ revealing nine-headed lambs and other Earth bound creatures as the means of our destruction/

The end of all humanity/when it slowly came/was beyond even the wildest of our imaginings in its subtle justice/

and materially and obviously alongside that it is difficult to ascertain exactly who had ignored whom for the past fifteen years of games with absence and presence /aspects were definitely and reciprocally turned to each other/the staring felt mutual/ although quite who was starer and who was staree was difficult to ascertain/

APRIL 15th /TIGHT THIN PALE GREEN BUDS AT THE END OF ALMOST EVERY GREY BROWN BRANCH OF THE HORSE CHESTNUT/

When had they arrived?/ It seemed an overnight occurrence/ surely they had not been there yesterday/ April 16th the pale green buds were burgeoning out/ almost bursting/ like fat leaf-filled plums/ How come I had never noticed this extraordinary process before?/April 17th/a smattering of the plum-like buds on the branch near the window, and on one other branch lower down the tree/in close to the trunk/had burst open into crumpled shiny bright green spikey leaves, still semi-furled/ April 18th A few more branches close into the trunk burst forth/ April 19th
wood pigeons perched on the branch outside the window/ feasting on the fat pale green buds/ Several more pairs of pigeons arrived on other branches/ April 21st the whole tree was covered in shiny spiky leaves/ just a few pale green plum shaped buds remaining here and there/ There were no pigeons to be seen/ April 22nd the horse chestnut is OUT in all her gloss and greenery/covered in new shiny/ hand-like leaves/ April 26th the leaves are getting bigger, hanging down in bunches of five from the ends of each branch/ May 1st there are narrow brown spikes sprouting out from the centre of each bunch of leaves/ May 5th the brown spikes have unfurled small branches, like little brown Christmas trees/May 12th
the brown spikes have grown to at least 6 inches long/they are all over the tree and each of their little branches has a brown curled bud at the end/A brown spike for every 5 leaves all over the tree/the leaves have lost their shine, they are a paler/ matte green now and much larger than when they first appeared/ each leaf about the size of my hand/ Still spiky and droopy though/ May 15th the spikes are unfurling into paler/pinker stalks/candelabra for dark pink buds/May 19th the buds are brimming open/deep pink on the outside and paler pink petals inside/ten or twelve on each stalk/erect like candelabra/ The tree has become a

carnival/a procession/ May 20th small green plum like fruit are forming at the base of each flower /June 1st the flowers are opening out on the spikes/heavier now/with petals unfurled and open/ June 6th Summer/

NOT ONLY WAS I ALONGSIDE THE HORSE CHESTNUT, WATCHING AND WAITING AND IDLING AND STARING, but the horse chestnut was also alongside me – so vibrantly and materially and obviously alongside that it was difficult to ascertain exactly who had ignored who for the past thirteen years – aspects were definitely and reciprocally turned to each other, and the staring felt mutual, although quite who was starer and who was staree was difficult to ascertain.

Have I told you that before? I think so/ this text is full of repetitions/ walking past the same trees/staring at the same park/saying the same words/repeating myself/re-meeting myself residual traces or a typing error/this is either some clever literary device or /

PLANE BLIGHT/OAK DECLINE/BEECH AND HORNBEAM WILT/HORSE CHESTNUT BLEEDING canker/ash die back and elm disease/a human lifetime's stretch of damage/ The trees are dying/ slowly dying as they grow/One thousand years up and quickly down/bleeding darkly from the middle/ rotten sap seeping out/

8 MILLION ASH TREES ALL AWAITING DIE-BACK/ does this include the lovely Rowan/I keep asking/does no-one answer because it is obvious/ the lovely mountain Ash with bright red berries in winter/ the last to leaf in spring/ the lovely Rowan/the national tree of Wales/a tree that bends and gnarls to westerlies /outlives hurricanes of tanker ripping strength and waits along the lanes to unfurl slowly out of moss-buttered banks into dark feathered

leaves and grey-black bark/can this strange disease that has crossed the North sea upon the feet of gulls and tourists Intend to destroy these friendly/grizzled hedgerow beasts/

HOW WILL OUR CHILDREN'S CHILDREN KNOW WHERE THEY ARE ON EARTH IF THE ROWANS ALL DIE BACK/will our hedgerows/like our high streets/become uniform/
straight-trunked mundane affairs/ will we import rows of slender Cyprus as well as killer diseases/
there is no cure for Ash die-back they say/ all 8 million are under threat/a holocaust/ but they do not speak about the Rowan/ the lovely Rowan/

THE ROWAN THAT STOOD ABOVE MY SWING WAS MY FIRST TREE FRIEND/I SAT FOR HOURS BENEATH HER/pushing to and fro/ her filigree/fern-like canopy protecting me from burning as I dreamed and swished/ I remember the noises in the garden /all the clanking and the creaking the night before my birthday/ and drawing back the curtains in the half-light I saw the swing my father was erecting at the bottom of the garden beneath the Rowan tree/

8 million Ash trees/we outnumber them 60 to 8, that's 7.5 to I/ we are no longer trying to save them/we cannot eradicate the die-back/ some will remain immune/ resistant to this plague/ Would they try to save us I ask/ some of them are over one thousand years old/what cure could they not find/those wizened elders/ my Rowan tree was young and slender-stemmed/ yet wise beyond her years and full of secrets/ She would have saved me/ we would have done anything for each other/ in the end I googled it/according to the forestry commission/the Rowan/ sometimes called the Mountain Ash/ belongs to the Sorbus species and is not/ strictly speaking/an Ash tree as such/the Ash trees belong to the Fraxinus species/

she will not die back my old friend/ I am not so distraught now/It is only the Ash trees /not my wizened beauties that are going to die/ I am saddened still/but feel relieved my inner landscape has escaped this culling/we will still have our lovely Rowan/how many million Rowan trees are there/how do they know there are 8 million Ash trees/do the Ash family fill in their annual census forms/Even If they do/I feel sure that the less orderly/Celtic-fringed Rowans do not/

DUTCH ELM FORMS ANOTHER BRANCH OF CHILDHOOD MEMORY/A VISION of the elm tree avenue beyond the old ruins disappearing one winter/ What other blights will blow in on the trade winds across these shores/Dutch elm/ Ash die-back/What other forces of destruction lie in future storms/What lurks in these early November gusts and blusters for the brave horse chestnuts outside my window in the park/They are all diseased it seems/some cancerous fungus has crept inside and is eating its way steadily outwards/ These prosperous post war years have brought with the a life timeline of tree diseases/ I was Born in 1954/ 1971 Dutch elm disease *ophiostoma nova-ulmi/* (tens of millions of elm trees) 1983 disease in Alders – *Phytophthoria*/1997 needle blight in Pine trees – *dothystroma*/2002 Beech tree disease – *Phytophthoria ramorum*/2004 Bleeding canker of horse chestnut/*Pseudamonas syringae* – (fewer than 2 million horse chestnuts) /2006 Beech and Hornbeam disease – *phytophthoria pseudo syringae/* 2010 – acute Oak decline and Plane blight/ 2012 Ash die back *Chalara fraxinea* (8 million trees)

THINGS ARE HOTTING UP/ I WORRY ABOUT OUR TREES/8 million native Ash trees subject to a Himalayan disease (bloody foreigners/UKIP is getting more and more votes)/And the 2 million horse chestnuts/ brought here from the Balkans in the 1500s by John Tradescant/the royal gardener/ in the early days of an empire upon which the sun never set/unknowingly uprooted and blighted/ like the Mayans/ falling in their thousands to a common

Spanish head cold/ empire and globe/how swiftly
exploration turns to exploitation/and the earth
cringes and crumbles
as we wreak this havoc on every shore/ now our Oak trees
are weeping/a dark weeping of the stem/and the London
Plane trees dropping their progeny/losing all new buds and
shoots as they grow/we have been slowly murdering our
trees all my life/but I have never watched a tree as closely
and precisely as I have watched the horse chestnut outside
my window in the park/she is my constant watchful
companion/we alternate staree and starer into each other's
parallel lives...

LAST NIGHT I DREAMT AGAIN OF
PEMBROKESHIRE/OF WALKING THE COASTAL
PATH/we were sitting by the copper mine just west of
Treginnis/ the sun in the west behind us/warming our
backs as we sat on the warm stone/Ramsey sound and the
island cliffs behind us/we have to watch the dog lest she
goes over to the mine shaft/a long drop that/

And then I remembered/
And wondered/How I'd got there/Had my limbs
restarted/rekindled themselves in this dream?/Or was this
just a memory of a dream from a life I no longer live?
I could have got there the other way/I suppose/
Over Treginnis and down the blackberry lane in a
wheelchair or something/
But in the dream I had got there unaided/leaning
Against the warm mossy stone/stone against the skin/just
like before all this/before all this/

When I woke the sun had risen in the west and was blasting this side of the park with light/the horse chestnut was bathed in a bright orange and pinkish light, the higher twiggy branches picked out, casting deep maroon filigree shadows on the glowing trunk/the dark green trunks of the lime trees a shadowy avenue behind/the park lit as if for a film set in the Louisiana bayou, not the cool grey skies of Northern Europe/we get this bright winter light and orange/pink sky quite often in these winter hills above the city/

[
[
]
]
]
]
] again
]
]

] often

] if not, winter/

]
]

remembering life in hospital/in the last days of the Bristol General /Bristol voices across the park/

Do you want me to get anything down ASDA lunchtime?
/I explained it to her when I got her dressed why she
couldn't have a pad in/ I'll just get her washed and do this/

I'm from the North Philippines – Mindanao and all the floods are in the south/ I'm going home for Christmas/I'll be alright/everyone is alright/It's alright in the North/I'm named Imelda after the president's wife/the one with all the shoes/ there are lots of girls my age named Imelda/I didn't used to like my name/She's not very popular/ it's all the corruption you know/but she did good things too/ corruption and lots of charity work/that was her pattern/ both sides to her/you know/but that's human beings for you/innit?/

This young woman said she's not having her grand-mother's clothes through her washing machine/ I got so annoyed I said/
I got a dog/ I put all his bedclothes through on a wash/
why can't she treat her grandma like I treats me dog?/
we've got a washing machine
In this hospital/for the people who ain't got no relatives an that/we wash their stuff/Bet they haven't thought about that in this new build/

Why am I not getting my brain into gear?
Why am I not walking down the ward?

Elsie has been groaning all night/she is all set this morning to groan her way through the day/Lyndy the housekeeper tells me about her friend who was diagnosed with cancer nine weeks ago and who died yesterday on New Year's eve/ [in Iran they have New Year's Eve on March 21st/that's our winter solstice/I'd be ready to start a new year then/Christmas/hibernation for three months/ New year/SORTED]/she died/Lyndy's friend/ having refused all treatments/she died in the hospital/where is the palliative care for Elsie?/Are you in any pain? /Is it your chest?/she takes no notice when the nurses ask her/ no responsibility for this dying state she is in/ I lie next to her wondering how much responsibility she took in her living/I have been quietly blaming the nurses and the unflinching ethics of the medical profession for the length and breadth of Elsie's dying/but this is Elsie's death and I am an uninvited witness/ I received no invitation to this wake/ I have spent three weeks in the bed beside her/now I am back in the ward as a witness to this death/ I have come back from my single cell/last week I lay wondering/ in my side room/whether Elsie had died/ in my two weeks away from the ward/but no/the nurses treat her with such tenderness/ I want to shout 'MORPHINE'/give her morphine/lots of morphine/more than she needs/ that's not fair/they are not allowed to do that/we await the house of lords report/Mary Warnock and her morals are not discussed in here/ Mavis and I discuss how we want and do not want to die/I talk about how my dogs were treated in the hours before their deaths/dignity/ Elsie is still groaning/she groaned right through our conversation/

BANANA BOARD/TRANSFERS FROM THE BED TO THE CHAIR AND BACK/SHUFFLE ALONG/lean forward over your feet/lift bum/position feet/hand on the edge of the board/right to the end/focus on where you are going/centre of gravity/not too far/where's your left arm?/

standing swap/push forward head over the rest/head over your feet/hand on the bar/pushing not pulling/esoteric knowledge this/

shuffling from the commode to the wheelchair/not that straightforward/ [ ] there little said [ ] and sideways movement/
where are you going?/where are my feet?/

One third of stroke patients will remain permanently disabled/which third will I be in?/ Nobody knows – they say/Nobody can tell – they tell me /you are making good progress/ this is a good sign/the earlier the progress/ the age of onset/ the steep curve at the beginning indicates a steep recovery/but does not predict anything/they cannot predict anything/this is the meaning of 'patient'/

RUTHIE PHONES/ SHE ASKS: 'BUT CAN YOU FEEL MOVEMENT? WILL YOU BE ABLE TO WALK SOON? Have you done any walking? What are they doing with you?' /

And I think: she wants me 'back to normal'/everybody is going for 'normal'/let's not have any changes here/let's not have any body changes/the half full cup means getting to 'normal'/ not embracing 'otherness' with grace/what if I am permanently altered by this? /is this different from the 'old Jane' I am beginning to sound like? /
last night I wiggled my left foot/only once/I could only do it once/ 'left foot wiggle!' I said/and it did/I moved on the right/ but the left was a poor imitation//I really had to think about it/it did not want to wiggle/whereas before wiggling would have been the order of the day/ 'come on pathways open up/find new routes/get that foot wiggling'/ it did not happen the next morning/

That night I heard the beating of the drums in the clubs down by the river/and I tried to tap my feet/I heard the sirens coming over the weighbridge/clumping and clanking their way across the city/the grey lady/ghost of the hospital/walks the fourth floor/according to local gossip handed down betwixt hospital staff and local Bedminster people/ they danced together on the hospital roof/the grey lady and the woman in the moon/

Miss Jenner had worked in a milliner's shop down Ashley hill once/she still liked hats/always wore a hat/even in the summer/woolly in the winter/and gloves/she liked gloves/ she had worn white silk gloves in the shop/going into the window/lifting out the fancy hats and veiling/her dad had been a builder/built most of the houses round the park/ by all accounts/she lost the house when he died/there'd been money before he died/but then they put her in a flat/ with a few sticks of furniture and well one thing had led to another/how it does/and here she was/everything she owned was in this trolley/she liked that/taking it all with you where you went/cardigans/she liked cardigans/always wore a few cardigans/useful items cardigans were/easy in the onning and offing/

PATIENT CONFIDENTIALITY/SUDDENLY THE CURTAINS GO UP ROUND MY BED/A CONVERSATION/ 'heard you talking to a person on the phone about a conversation you heard the nurses having'/ she says/'that breaches patient confidentiality'/But I'm a patient/ I've not contracted to work for UHBT/I see and hear things about which/as a human being/ I have a view/ this is all being debated about in the news/assisted death/ it is interesting to hear what the nurses think/what the housekeepers think/ putting curtains around does not give privacy you know/do you seriously think the other patients and their visitors do not see and hear what goes on?/

But I feel vulnerable/I lack the sense of self and confidence in my opinions I had in my life outside these walls/
Sweetheart/ my loverly/ sweets/my luvver/ darling/ flower/here my love/what do you want to be called Harry or Henry? /I likes sweetheart best love/
alright sweetheart can you pick up that left foot?/ I can hear you dragging it down the ward/

It's only the left side left hanging/ the right is alright/ and my memory's scattered/ so this is a stroke/
what's the name of the prime minister?/ David Cameron I reply/perfect – he smiles/If you think he's perfect you've got no business working for the NHS I spit out/ what day is it today he asks –warily/ November 18th, 2011, I retort/

Mind if I do your obs? / Mind you the machine's playing up today/ sometimes it works/
sometimes it doesn't/no blood pressure today? / perhaps I'm dead/ perhaps you are/ No/ it's okay I've got one: 110/68/ that's okay/and the temperature as well/ thirty-eight degrees that's okay then/that's okay/

/WHERE AM I GOING? / I DON'T KNOW WHERE I'M GOING/ we've come to take you home/home to your home/(Mavis chucks her earplugs in the bin)/they wipe her name off the ward list/it is as if Daisy was never here/ how do they do this?/making such connection and then so quickly parting from her/she's not gone home to her old home/says the sister/it's not such a good home/not one of the best/when she's left they take down the cards from behind her locker/dear mum/dear mum/ dear mum/ from when she was 91/but they never came to see her/ the children and grandchildren/just the one son came to see dear mum/and we held their feelings for them/ on the ward/ we are tearful in our goodbyes/

NOW I HAVE MOVED TO A ROOM OF MY OWN/ NO MORE EARPLUGS/THE SIDE WARD/no sagas to record here/more introspection and rumination/ I am getting the hang of this one-handed life/I have just been up to chat to Mavis/

I have been measured/ I need a wheelchair that is eighteen inches across/twenty inches long and eighteen inches tall/

I'm going home on Christmas day/they are going to decide on Friday/ Saturday is Christmas eve and then I might be going home/

YOU ARE GOING TO DO A STANDING SWAP/ HANG ON TO THAT BAR IN FRONT OF YOU AND WE ARE GOING TO TAKE THE WHEELCHAIR AWAY BEHIND YOU AND SWAP IT FOR THE COMMODE/so/meanwhile you are going to be balancing your weight between your left side and your right/

Half the day has gone/what have I been doing?
Waking/peeing/washing/breakfast/teeth/ pulling myself right up to look in the mirror/ my hair needs doing badly/
Time spent in the company of nobody who loves you/they care for you/ this is what it must be like in 'care'/ they come and go on their shifts/ I am in the care of the NHS/ love/ flower/petal/queen/darling/and then I am writing/there is plenty of time to write/I watch daytime TV before lunch/ lunch is noon/we chat around the table/ Simon has a sense of humour/so has Mavis/thank God/ and Kelly/she's as bright as a button/and now I am back to my cubicle/
And sometimes/like Susie with Daisy/some of this care transforms to love/at night Susie sits with Daisy who is frightened/and spoons hot chocolate into her mouth, which Daisy expects and anticipates/ she feels loved/

[And fucking hell/she'll do the drugs for 2 hours and then she'll have her break/fucking hell/]

They do not wait/like me/ for visits from their loved ones/I am being looked after/but I know this is temporary/while my loved ones prepare for new lives looking after someone like me/what if they refused?/ his wife refused/ not my Sarah/my lovely Sarah who comes nearly every day/these visits are like liquid love/ love in action/

[We are going to assess her capacity/what's her capacity/ he asks the physio students/]

the midline/when it feels like I'm veering towards the left I am actually standing upright/this is the first time in my life I've ever been accused of leaning to the right/

PATIENCE/THIS IS THE MEANING OF PATIENTS/
WE WAIT TO BE GOT UP/
washed/dressed/toileted/breakfasted/patiently we wait (except for Mr G.) /waiting for people/waiting for transport/waiting for my turn/life in the fast lane has been overturned/interrupted/

Waiting for Sarah/waiting for Sarah to come/cards/ messages/books/people send gifts and cards and Sarah covers the wall and the locker with these tokens/ colours that contradict the institutional ugliness of hospital walls and floors/

Where am I? shouts Daisy/ what am I doing here? Are my family downstairs?
[on the women's ward most patients have been in once or twice before/ they are all in their 80s and 90s/ third or second stroke/vascular dementia/ all sorts/ the men are younger/60s and 70s/ young Winston is the talk of the wards/ he is forty/ I am no longer the baby at 57/driving along the M4/ he was lucky to be alive/he made it to the hard shoulder/no-one was hurt/Mary Anne has lost everything down her left side/sight/hearing/breathing/I AM LUCKY]

FIRST OF ALL DONNA ASKS SALLY TO GO DOWN TO THE KITCHEN AND GET A SIDE SALAD/ she refuses and says / I'm not a domestic/they argue/then Mavis asks: Can I go now please? / Lena says: No/ You can't go back until all the patients have finished their food and their teas and coffees/that's the rule/I ask: Can I go to the toilet please? / Lena says: yes/ in a minute/just wait for everybody to finish/I say: that's a new rule isn't it?/ Lena: no that's always been the rule/ we have to wait for everybody to go back/we have to make sure you are safe/what are you doing with that left hand?/ we all have to stick by the rules/
Mavis: I just want to go back/
Jane: Mavis is twice your age Lena, Its really rude to treat older people like children/
Lena: well I'm sorry if you think we are patronising/
Jane: not 'we' it's just you I'm talking to...

The 'w' word. Why does nobody say 'walk?'
'walking is the last thing/your ultimate outcome/does she mean this sarcastically, as in 'walking is the last thing you should be aiming for' or seriously as in 'walking is the

very end of your therapeutic journey?' walking. We are all obsessed with walking/will I walk/how far?/ how long?/

TODAY IT WAS CHAOTIC IN THE PARK.
IT WAS THE HOTTEST DAY OF THE YEAR SO FAR.

Why?
Why these narratives? Why this excessive proliferation of pathways across the landscape of the park, and if there are going to be three (as opposed to four or ten million), why a murder mystery; an ethnography and a life story, and why are these narratives mediated by and negotiated around a tree? I have a preference for writing in three parallel voices (Sakellariadis, et al., 2008; Speedy, 2005) and although a simultaneity of ten million stories thus far would be nearer to the excess, loss and chaos that I would like to create I have interrupted my attempt to manicure the ten million into three clear bordered storylines, without wandering too far into the territories of 'getting lost'. I am writing in what Lather (2007) described as the post-critical era, playing amidst the 'ruins' of methodology and refusing to be 'constrained by the dominant notions of truth', to which end a text that blurs and brushes edges between image and writing, fact and fiction, and research and novel writing genres – and positions a horse chestnut tree as one of , if not *the* main character and narrator, sits comfortably with the constantly interrupted / disrupted world I find myself inhabiting. I am grateful to Jane Reece (2015/forthcoming) and Norman Denzin (1997) for bringing the similarities and proximities of qualitative research and detective work into play with each other and perhaps bringing my post retirement ambitions to write crime novels and my previous post as a professor of qualitative inquiry into juxtaposition and conversation with each other/
All the narratives that make up this text are woven into the fabric of the park that I look out on and are made visible by my newly found practices of staring.... Not watching or observing you understand, but ***staring.*** Staring is not

at all polite. Staring is a hardened penetrating practice of looking that brings to light the dark spaces beneath the trees and the traces of spectres in the shadows of the park. The body in the paddling pool was made apparent through my reveries and my practices of staring, in the same way as the cankerous/cantankerous nature of the horse chestnut tree became transparent. Long hours of looking, longing and belonging gave birth to the life stories of the park, of which I am one/

I did not loiter in the park, conducting interviews as is considered commonplace, even common sense in social science research/I did not listen to the conversations I had captured on my pocket digital recorder, nor did I transcribe them thence into written text/

I listened to the park on a daily basis, mingled with my own recent memories, my senses attuned to familiar rhythms and songs/I recorded the park's sounds and silences, inhabited and otherwise, on my iPad in image and text/ I am complicit/ I am both formed by and forming/becoming in this/ situated/this text is neither outside nor inside my experience/we write each other/

> I lost track of time, becoming lost in that other way that isn't about dislocation but about the immersion where everything else falls away.
>
> (Solnit, 2005, p. 36)

My staring proved to be a different form of listening – the kind of listening that inscribes and scorches voices into the surfaces of the park and wrings hidden and long forgotten voices out of the trees and out of the red earth and brown Bristol rock beneath/ visceral/visual sharp-edged listening/

Third plateau

We rattled through the wrought iron gates/doc

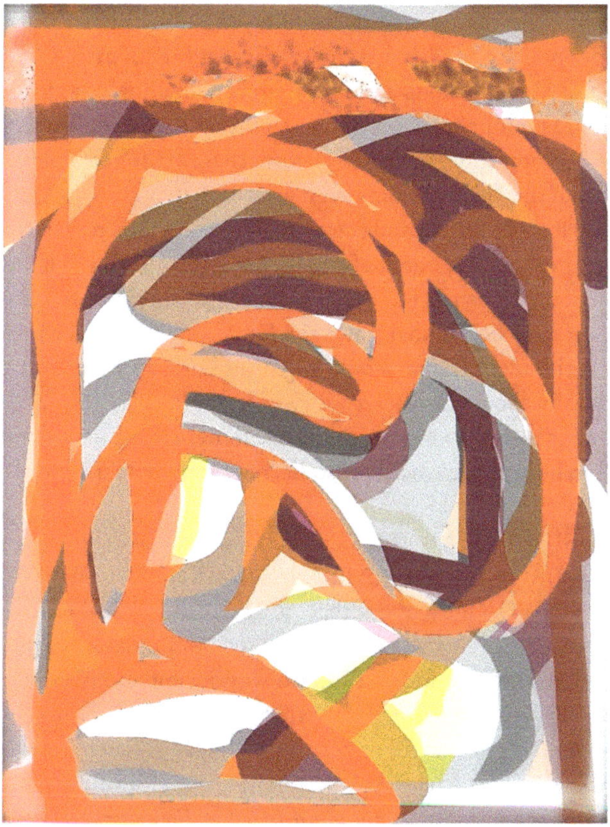

horse chestnut and me – entanglement

Starring at the Park: A Poetic Autoethnographic Inquiry, Jane Speedy, 93–115.

WE RATTLED THROUGH THE OLD IRON GATES INTO AN OLD STONE BUILDING LIKE A WORKHOUSE.../MY GOD, they are taking me to the Bristol workhouse

/we clatter into the cobbled yard/I am lifted out of the ambulance and bundled across the yard, past the lit up glass booth of the night porter's lodge/it is cold/at the other side of the yard I can see the tall Bristol brownstone buildings rising up/ the top floor of the structure rises in a dark, blackened silhouette against the fading sky/the building appears to be burnt out: bombed, perhaps, or maybe there has been a fire?/they are taking me into a bombed-out workhouse building and along a corridor that smells of lavender polish and disinfectant with a faint hint of urine/ we go up in a large noisy lift and along another, similarly smelling corridor/this is another hospital/a poor people's hospital/we enter a ward and I am stretchered up onto a bed opposite the nurse's station/there are two of them: Kathy and Lauren/ if this text reinvents itself with each new reading, as well as carrying with it the imprints and traces of all the previous readings and writings/ other names, once thought of and thence discarded remain under erasure on top of the crossings out beside Kathy and Lauren who were once Karen and Laura and before that Katie and Lorna/ is what I am writing true or is it fuzzy at the edges where people might get hurt? / I get up, scattering words into the sky above the trees/those words might be as good as these/ I have a sense of us interweaving our thoughts in these inhabited silences (Mazzei, 2007) in between us/these prosodic/poetic spatial /silent features/

LEFT SIDE/I HAD THIS WEAKNESS ON MY LEFT SIDE/A LACK OF SENSATION/ NO SENSE/ I DID NOT STOP TO WONDER about this/ it was how it was when I fell/ I adapted/if the left arm could not lift me up/I'd have to use the right/ instant adaptation/ I did no wondering about the oddness of this situation/ or about what this might be or mean or how this might be named or described simply got on with being (for this was truly what Virginia Woolf [2002]) would describe as a 'moment of being'/a moment of what Deleuze would call haecceity or 'just thisness' (Davies & Gannon, 2013)/ I was as one with my surroundings and blended effortlessly/ cyborg-like/ with the laptop in my hand and the carpet beneath my body/adapting in the moment/

]
]
]

]
]
]

[this

moment]

[

THIS WAS AN A C T U A L EXPERIENCE OF LIVING IN THE MOMENT WITH NO DESIRE TO SEARCH FOR A STORY TO LIVE BY/ through or about what was happening/ this was an unstoried moment like no other I remember, a non-discursive moment in the life of a multiply-storied, highly discourse-ridden woman/the stroke, like being born perhaps, was a purely visceral, felt experience/I had no words or stories to describe it at the time/ PRE-LINGUISTIC OR POST-LINGUISTIC/the words are only coming now/ Later in hospital, when Cindy sent me pastels, I could draw it/ I could get

an image of it in my mind's eye, but I had no words for it – and afterwards, finding myself lying on the floor, I just began to adapt/without thought/not a flicker/extraordinary/]

A NEW WAY OF SEEING/ STARING INTO SPACE/I LOOKED DOWN ON THE STRETCH OF NON-SLIP GREY MOTTLED NON SLIP HOSPITAL FLOORING/ITWAS A MATTE, MULTI-COLOURED, MARBLE-EFFECT SORT OF FLOORING/ A resin, perhaps, that they had poured onto the surface of the ward. It went a little bit up the wall – about three inches and then stopped/ every day the furniture was moved and the floor behind the bed was mopped/ it was clinically, brutally clean/ looking the other way, there were white ceiling tiles – a pattern of lights embedded/the one above Blanuk was not working/ that became my homing beacon as I drifted off at night / my way home marked by the non-lit light/ I spent long days staring at that floor and long nights non-lighting my way back to my bed/I had a locker, an armchair and a bed/ this marked out my territory/

Some other inmates had wheelchairs or Zimmer frames at the end of their beds but I, at first, had no such indication of mobility or of a world beyond my little section of the ward/this was my world/I inhabited this space and others visited, or occasionally intruded upon me in it/ my experience was very visual and visceral – an entirely new way of seeing/ that piece of non-slip flooring came under scrutiny in a way that no

o
t
h
e
r

f
l
o
o
r

h
a
d

been examined by me before – every working brain cell was focused on the floor – it became a practice of staring – not looking, observing or watching, but of staring. I was idling, my eyes

wandering around the room and then I would lose myself in the patch of floor, staring into it, confronting and confronted by its smooth matte surface – national health service non-slip flooring

Staring at the park became a daily dreamscape practice. As for Walter Benjamin (1999) and the surrealists, the landscape before me took on a dreamlike quality/ I was sharply focussed, but I was not always gazing or attending outwards, often my vision blurred as I looked. I stared 'too hard'. I was looking 'too far'

m
u
s
t

b
e

s
u
b
j
e
c
t

to this kind of scrutiny daily. It's a wonder I didn't wear a hole in it with my gaze/ it felt like a boring process, boring down through the flooring into a

> When we 'see' a landscape we situate ourselves in it.
>
> (Berger, 1967, p. 70)

practice of internal reverie that brought forth the spectral traces of former occupants and inhabitants/ this was the practice of staring that I was to take home with me and take to the lush, verdant, multi-peopled scenes in the park across from my bedroom window/ at first it all seemed so confusing after the order of the hospital, all these lives, not seemingly connected to each other, crossing over and tangling in the park. I was confused until I found my bearings/my horse chestnut and my focus/ in the hospital, staring had come easily/ looking at the park, I had to learn to focus again – staring is a very different visual practice from watching/

AN OPEN SPACE/ QUESTIONING CONVERSATIONS/ MEMORIES FLUID AND SHAPES SHIFTING/ I am writing from memories and imaginings/material witnessed/ material remembered and material imagined whilst staring at the park/ not everything that came to mind whilst I was staring at the park /but a lot of it/ these memories and imaginings are more like distillations of experience over time than carefully selected extracts/ thus memories/ experiences and imaginings are all fluid and shifting/they leak sideways/slip about and overlap/ this does not make them not true or less real/these may not be confessional realist tales/ but they all have truth and integrity/are all sedimented in the mind/ assemblages of the spirit/of the park that I see stretched out before me both geographically/ from my bedroom window/ and psychically throughout the landscapes of my mind/in some senses I bored my way through that hospital floor right out into this park/ but by these assemblages around which the rest of life silts up/the memories and imaginings are not spaced evenly by time's compass points/ but by accumulations in the moment:

I bored my way through that hospital floor right out into this park

> *These were the moments other things clustered around, when life stepped out of its rhythm and lingered a while on the shore.*
>
> (McCleen, 2013, p. 1037)

WHAT CAN YOU SEE THROUGH YOUR FOG AND FATIGUE? What can you make out by screwing up your eyes and bringing the people and the park into focus? Can you see the Victorian park-makers laying out the pattern of paths? Can you see the wreckage of the bomber that crashed here in the war? Can you hear the sounds of the bombs that landed nearby in Leopold and Walsingham roads? It is all there beneath the layers of Greenery/ silted up in the wooded Shadows behind the bowling green/Not so Anne Carson's red-winged Geryon cowering in brilliant epic tales ancient and modern/ other winged creatures lurk in more prosaic climes and moments/Can you hear the sounds of the M32 down in the eastern valley? Is this an inner or outer landscape? an inner motorway/an outer dreamscape/ uncertainty and gravity remain/ I know nothing of the electro-magnetic fields that keep us on this planet/and yet, despite a lack of comprehension of the laws of physics/I am here/I know little of the ancient laws of poetics/and yet I write these words/

MY FAVOURITE COUPLE ENTER THE PARK FROM THE NORTH/ HER LONG HAIR SWAYING IN THE LIGHT BREEZE/it is November/ but sunny and crisp/autumn is late this year/ the horse chestnut an inner golden brown/an outer green/they are holding hands/ they are always holding hands / they stride down the avenue of plane trees with their German shepherd at their heels/ he has his dog walking rucksack/he always has his dog walking rucksack/ a metal drinking bowl tied on at the back/ they are wearing hats/they are always wearing hats/even in summer/

SCREAMING AT SARAH/IT JUST APPEARS TOTALLY OUT OF THE BLUE – A FULL-ON RAGE, LIKE A TORNADO/whipped up from nowhere/not remotely in the forecast, and lasts about half an hour all told/'I'm going to leave you if you carry on like this for the next twenty years' she says, but I scarcely hear her/I am at full throttle by now, steaming ahead/the last full-blown ripsnortwarbler was in the car, parked outside Lloyds' bank/ We had not brought the blue badge/ it had been left at home in the pocket of/'well this is why I always put everything I need in my handbag' I yell/'you take the piss out of me for this handbag fetish I've developed/ but everything I need is always in there/keys, phone, iPad, glasses/ disabled?/I couldn't spend my time traipsing round the house looking for all my stuff every time I wanted to go out/I needed it all in/blue badge/it's all in the bag/and when one of you borrows my stuff and doesn't put it back, I could scream'/ I was screaming by now at the top of my voice/I had made myself hoarse within seconds/I went on and on and on/I was incensed/How could she be so stupid?/ Didn't she know I was my handbag/right where I'd put it/in the end she just turned the radio up full blast and drove home with gritted teeth and a grim expression/ the following day, I made her drive me down into the city centre in the Christmas traffic to the co-op bank/ when we got there I discovered that I had not brought my chequebook/I sat in silence all the way back home/

THIS NARRATIVE ETHNOGRAPHIC ACCOUNT OF LIFE IN AND AROUND ST. ANDREWS PARK BRISTOL WAS CONDUCTED OVER A PERIOD OF 25 MONTHS THROUGHOUT 2012–2014/ according to the Oxford English dictionary ethnography is the scientific description of peoples and cultures and their customs, habits and mutual differences/ originating with anthropological studies of 'exotic' peoples, ethnography has been taken up by a variety of social science disciplines and is now widely used by sociologists, educationalists, geographers and many others in the study of everyday lives/ethnographies seek to form an in-depth or 'thick' (Geertz, 1977) description of everyday life and aim not just to describe events and experiences but also to construct explanations or 'webs of meaning' (Geertz, 1977) description out of human endeavours and encounters with their environments/ thus, in conducting this reflexive and iterative study I hope to 'exoticise' not only my own life, but the lives of those around me who use the park that my own house overlooks and their webs of interrelationship with each other; the circus school students/the yummy mummies/the eco-warriors/the dog walkers/the dogs/the neighbourhood residents/the footballers/ the pre-school children/the school children/the hoodies/the students/the festival and party goers/the picnickers/the travellers/the tai chi practitioners and other 'keep fit' doers/the café owners and workers/the drummers and musicians/the joggers/the park workers/the homeless bench-dwellers/ the paperback book readers/the courting couples/the community police/the drug users/the drug dealers/ all these people have stories to tell about the

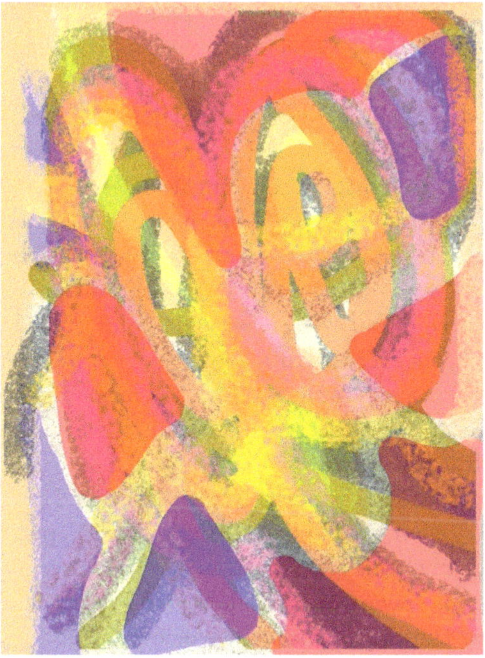

trails of tape

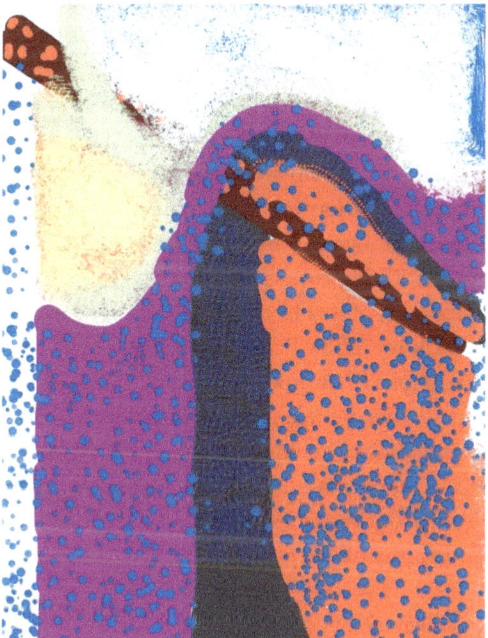

whispering bats

interchange between their lives and the park/stories in which the park itself/ the trees themselves, in particular/as well as the story-tellers/have some agency/I am already, as a local resident living in a house overlooking the park, a *participant* in the setting under investigation/I became, albeit unintentionally, an *observer* of the life of the park when I returned home my long stay in a local hospital stroke rehabilitation unit at the beginning of 2012/I had lived overlooking the park for the previous thirteen years and was a member of a number of the categories of park user listed above: I had walked my dog in the park and taught my child to ride a bike in it; but had never before had the time or cause to systematically study the everyday life of the park that I now had, sat in my bedroom every morning, staring out at the everyday vistas before me/prior to having my stroke, the park had formed a picturesque backdrop to my busy life, this was a nice part of Bristol to live in, and it was engaging to have so much activity going on outside my front door/the view from the living room of the horse chestnut tree and park beyond it was better than most inner city views, but beyond this sense of a backdrop to my 'real life' which went on inside my home and in my work at the University, the park had little impact/I became drawn into the park as a result of my developing relationship with the horse chestnut opposite my window and as a result of my morning cups of tea, drunk whilst sitting in the armchair beside my bed/I had often had tea in bed with my partner in the past, but these days I had much more time to sit and watch the comings and goings in the park outside and was not so intent and focussed on getting ready for the 'real' business of my life and work/staring at the park became a morning ritual for me/staring at the park became the 'real' business of my life: not only staring at the horse chestnut tree, but at all the people engaging in their morning rituals: the park workers collecting litter and emptying the bins; the joggers; the dog walkers; the secondary school students in their uniforms with big rucksacks of books on their backs, some on bikes, others on skateboards, others in clusters, walking; parents and children walking across the park to Sefton Park Primary school/drawing from Myerhoff's anthropological emphasis on 'making the familiar unfamiliar' (1982, pp. 1–35) whilst studying her own people; I began to study the familiar view and activities of the park as if making fieldnotes for an ethnographic study/I was, to quote Bourdieu (1988, p. xi), 'exoticising' my own 'domestic', using staring over a cup of tea out of my bedroom window as my method

/why an ethnography of the park?

/why now?/

why am I doing all this?/

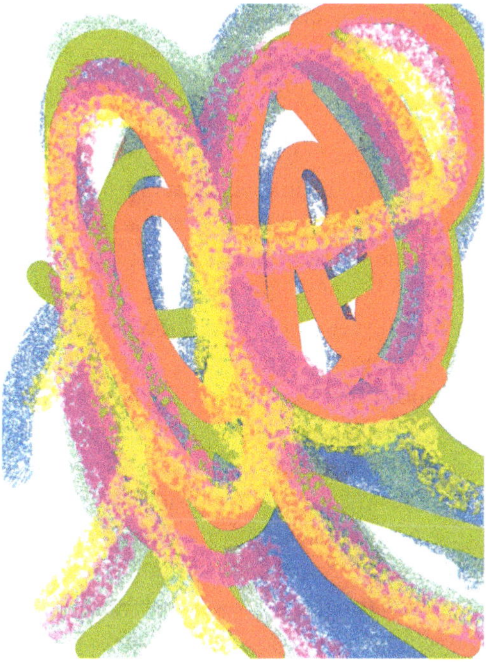

trails of tape 2

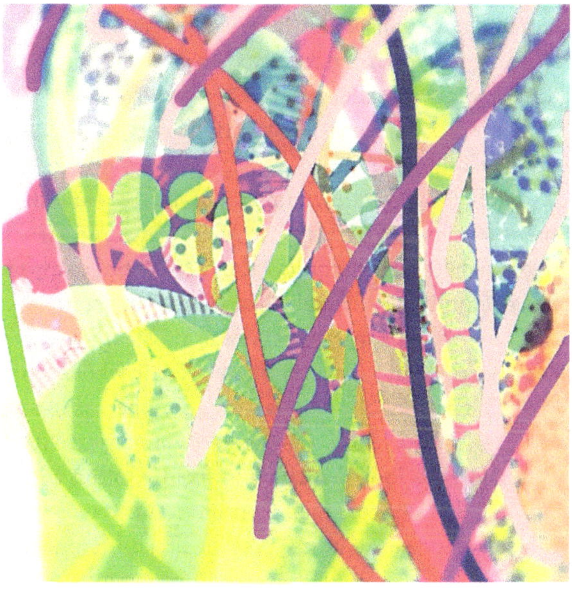

residual traces in the grass

partly to make some sense of my own recent life, through the prism of my past, and partly to give something back to the neighbourhood and city in which I live: to weave some webs of meaning into the landscape of St. Andrews Park, so that this neighbourhood can see itself reflected in the mirror I have held up to it/as a recently and prematurely retired academic, I have spent a great deal of my professional life immersed in one kind of ethnographic study or another, indeed, my life's work in both research and practice has been about bringing to light the extraordinariness that often lies buried in the stories that people assume are of no consequence and speak only of the mundane and everyday/I see myself as an excavator of forgotten, half-remembered and rarely told tales/I hope that this inquiry will bring some insights into the diverse communities that live around and use St. Andrews Park/I hope to work to bring together stories and images of people whose lives cross over and bump up alongside each other's everyday/as they cross and re-cross the park – weaving collective patterns into the environment – like 'songlines' – into each other's lives/ I hope this work allows a local knowledge to emerge that permits the people and communities to understand themselves a little better and for new local insights to evolve/I also hope to discover something of myself, for myself, as I sit in my eyrie bedroom, observing the life of the park /negotiating my own life/the more I learn about the park, the more I learn about myself/I have spent a great deal of time over the past 18 months staring into space and have consequently learnt a great deal about the art of staring/ every morning I have turned towards the park with my cup of tea in my hand, a) to witness what occurs...
[I am no longer so sure of the distinctions between ethnography and neighbourhood gossip]
or, b) iPad in hand, to set down images of the trees and the landscape/
these interventions into park life, these drawings and these acts of staring, are not incidental methods of inquiry/ they are central to my purpose/this whole study has been filtered through the prism of my stare: the insights are 'my' sights and come from a woman who was a former starer, now turned staree/ when I now go over into the park in my electric wheelchair or walking slowly with my stick, I am the one who is stared at, whereas in my bedroom eyrie, it is I who stare/ up here I am the starer/ I am not watching, you understand: I choose to *stare* (to look directly and fixedly; often with a wide-eyed gaze: Oxford online dictionary) and it is through this staring as method that I propose to make some sense of my present life, a life only a short time ago so

busy, hugely vital and active, now continuing with my left side damaged and weak/I do not sit here all the time, staring, but maintaining this daily ritual of staring out at the park, watching and befriending the horse chestnut tree, has made the most difference /this single daily act of communion with the park and those in it has connected me far more with my locality and community than anything else I have done for the past thirteen years of living here and, on a daily basis, getting into my car, parked outside in the street, and driving off down the road to the University/

THE STROKE A TURNING POINT IN MY EVERYDAY LIFE/A DISJUNCTURE IN MY ONGOING NARRATIVE /I lived in and walked the world/ trailing my various possible deaths/ up until the stroke/ dreamlike/ I had lived just outside the shadow of death/ dying – like ageing – happened to others/ now I live with defractions/ recollections/manifestations of people scraping my body off the floor and bundling me down the stairs/
I experience a new fragility and vulnerability/Bristol's uneven pavements – hitherto home territory – present new hazards/ crowds of young people milling around in the street seem dangerous/ frail now and unsure of my footing/ I rewrite my future every day according to my altered memories/ my spoiled identity and broken, creaky body parts/ I have been interrupted/

Luke made a bob or two on the side selling ketamine and home-grown skunk from his bench/near the Maurice road entrance/he wasn't exactly a dealer/ more personal use/and a little bit over/ (if this was Under Milkwood he'd be 'no good boyo')/ none of the hard stuff/ just his own skunk and a few bought-on ketamines for the students/no harm done/ there was some kid had a few psychotic episodes/ down at the Poly/nothing to link things to him though and nothing you could call statistically significant/ he bought the K's from old Grant down at the caff and sold them on for a bit of a mark up/ but it was the skunk that he made his real money on. Ever since he went hydroponic in the attic, he'd never lost a plant and they paid good money for it up in the park/ they even bought the extra large papers for a fiver/(a fiver, no kidding)/there was a real market for his stuff up in the park/last weekend there was a queue forming at the bench before he'd even got there

SHE HAD OFTEN FLOWN IN HER DREAMS/ SHE HAD BEEN FLYING ALL HER LIFE / but dream sequence flying hardly did justice to the real experience/ that moment of flinging herself off the window sill, wings outspread/ that moment of soaring up into the westerly wind/ she never knew quite what to do with her hands and arms and experienced a surfeit of upper body limbs as she crossed them in front of her – the position she had taken up in her primary school nativity play/ a position she had not had to call on in over fifty years/

THAT DAY I MISSED ANDY SPARKSE'S[1] WORKSHOP/ AFTER the flu jab the fog descended again cutting me off/adrift from myself and others/ my ears closed down/and a dull engine room throb presided over brain operations /heavy-limbed and weak-bladdered/ I heaved myself around at home/ slug-like and bedraggled/ unbothered about changing my socks/I stayed in my pyjamas all day and all night/how do I explain why I am not going to the workshop? how do I describe this layer of fatigue weighing in amongst the usual fog?/

I send them an e-mail saying I am tired describing myself as a 'poor old bat'/I briefly consider wheeling myself in, But then have an image of sitting at the back on my travelling commode because the disabled loo is too far away/even by myself, in the privacy of my own mind's eye/ my neck and cheeks blotch up at the thought/ 'she used to be a professor here, poor old bat/ but then she had a stroke/ and her oomph went out'/

I missed Tim Ingold too/despite his having written the defining guide to the paths across the park (Ingold, 2007)/ I wanted to ask him about the paths we could no longer see/ the coffin trails and the path across to the burial barrows in Baddock wood/ and the figures clad in roughly woven broadcloth garments/but perhaps the fact that he is interested in what he would call the 'dynamics of pedestrian movement' (Ingold, 2007, p. 152) would have been enough to attract and call him over to my window on the park /

SHE REACHED ACROSS THE PAPERS ON HER DESK FOR THE ASSIGNMENTS ON THE TOP OF THE PILE. THE UNIVERSITY HAD GONE OVER THAT YEAR TO AN EXCLUSIVELY DIGITAL HAND-IT-IN AND MARK-IT SYSTEM, a method much-loved by the course administrators and departmental managers. Abbi preferred to print her own student's work out on paper, read it and scrawl all over it in green ink, over lunch in one of the local cafes – ideally accompanied by a large glass of Montepulciano d'Abbbruzzo or an equivalently soft deep red. Hers was a method of marking deeply discouraged by her more 'quality-assurance' obsessed colleagues, as she left no digital trail. "Dr Taylor appears not to communicate any feedback to her students" was the only comment she had received from the last faculty board – which had now been renamed the faculty assembly (Fac-Ass for short), but fulfilled the same dysfunctions it had always done. Her protestations about a lack of recognition for the copious notes she wrote to her students and the more intimate relationship she felt these hand-written exchanges created, had fallen on stony ground. She had been taken aside by the graduate dean and assured that nobody objected to her hand-written notes, just as long as she copied everything they contained out onto the computer system as well.

Today she wanted to make some inroads into marking the auto-ethnography assignments from the doctoral programme. She grabbed the first six or seven papers and stuffed them into her shoulder bag before locking her office and striding off down the fourth floor corridor towards the lifts.

Abbi Taylor lectured in Education at the 'old' university in the centre of the city. This was her first job in Academia. She had come here about ten years ago, straight from her previous post as head of history in a local comprehensive school, where she had acted as an associate tutor to the university, supporting student teachers on their placements in her school. She had never previously conceived of herself as an academic of any sort, or had any ideas about an academic career, but she had gradually become interested in the work her colleagues at the university were doing, and after her appointment as a history

WATCHING A LITLE TODDLER IN
A RED JUMPSUIT
Learning to walk in the park
Maintaining his perpendicularity against
All odds and species.
Standing on two legs and moving
forwards –
Really going for it
In the perpendicular –
What an odd species!

Watching him surrounded by dogs of all
sizes in the park/
The four legged confidence of the dogs/
The two legged doggedness of the
toddler/
Determined to emulate the
Perpendicular adults/
He shows none of my hesitancy
As he teaches himself to walk/
Mimicking his parents he is
Strutting out/
One foot
Then another –
Off all fours and straight up –
Perpendicular in the winter wind/
Does he have to remember
To bend his knee/
I wonder/
As I watch
His faltering progress/

His pace is faster and
Gait is stronger and braver
In a day/
Than mine has become after a year of
this –

All pathways open
He skips across the grass –
Thoroughly human/
Perpendicular/

education lecturer, had gone on to take an increasing interest in the research aspects of the job, becoming less and less involved as the years went by in the practices of school teaching.

Martha cycled almost everywhere in the hilly city, but she did tend to get off her bike and push it up the pavement in Park street and today's climb up to the top of the hill was no exception. She slowed down her pace every now and then to peer into the myriad Park street cafes that lined her route and see if anybody she knew was sitting in the window, having a late coffee or an early lunch. She had got as far as Goldbricks, more than half way up, when she caught sight of Abbi tucking into the 'risotto of the day' and a glass of red. She banged on the window, startling her friend, who, looking up suddenly, knocked red wine all over the papers she was reading.

Martha couldn't hear clearly through the thick plate glass of the window, but she understood exactly what it was that Abbi was muttering as she rummaged through her large shoulder bag, searching for tissues to mop up the wine that was dripping off the papers and the table, down into her lap. Martha swiftly turned and chained her bike up to the nearest lamp-post. She knew she didn't really have the time to stop and chat because she was already a little late for the Arts Faculty Graduate Studies committee (known colloquially as Ars-Fac), but she felt that she could hardly just continue pushing her bike up the hill as if all this rumpus had not just occurred, or that it was nothing to do with her.

'Oops, sorry ducks' she declared jauntily, deciding to brazen it out as she entered the cafe, striding straight past Abbi, up to the counter.

'Let me get you another one...' she called back over her shoulder.

'Two large red wines please and a chocolate chip brownie...' She said to the barman

'I'm not stopping for long' Martha explained as she plonked herself down in front of Abbi. 'Just time before the faculty meeting to down a few essential supplies. Do you want some company or are you in the middle of some dreadful marking?'

'Both' said Abbi as she moved the papers to one side 'as in I both *have* to mark these assignments and also *desperately* need saving from them. This whole pile of essays is so heavily biased towards the weepier side of 'auto' and so light on its take up of the 'ethno' that I'm dreading what's going to happen now that I've used all my tissues, mopping up this wine. How's life in arts and farts?

'Well, Film Studies is as up its own arse as ever' said Martha, 'But Classics and Ancient History seem to have got a bit of a grip on the real world. They've got a new Prof. who keeps quoting chunks of Heroditus's critique of the restructuring of the Roman army to the Dean.... Not that I think it'll make any difference....'

Martha was working as a temporary research assistant in the department of Film and Television studies whilst finishing her doctoral thesis: a post structuralist, feminist critique of the role of the supporting female love object in television detective programmes, with special reference to central television's 38-episode adaption of Colin Dexter's 'Inspector Morse' books. Martha herself had no particular interest in Inspector Morse, but as the central character in the books was named after Lord Morse, a retired banker and chancellor of the university, she had discovered that she could get a substantial top-up bursary added to her research council funding if she included some 'special references' to the eponymous Morse series.

SCOSSI MET THE OTHER TWO THROUGH LIVING IN THE LITTLE HOUSE that sat between theirs, on the North side of the park. She and Abbi had been neighbours for a few years now and she was the Taylor house's number one baby and dog sitter. She had come across Martha a year or so ago, down at the bottom of the front steps, filling her recycling bins with old copies of 'Spare Rib'

"you don't want to throw them away darlin' ....priceless antiques they'll be in a year or so" She remembered yelling down the steps.

"Well I was going to take them over to the women's archive, but I gather they've been closed down ".

"bloody government. Close you down soon as look at you, those buggers. If you don't want em, I'll take em in for you, for now" Scossi offered. And promptly knelt down beside the bin to scoop up the Spare Ribs, carefully sorting them out from the rest of the bits of old leaflet and back copies of the Guardian.

'thanks. d'you want some help, there's rather a lot of them, almost the complete works", said Martha with pride." My mum had them delivered every month all through my childhood. I've kept them for years, but I'm having a major clearout and I've made a big decision.....everything I don't actually read any more has to go!"

"blimey if I did that there'd be nothing left' said Scossi, looking both impressed and aghast.

And thus began a friendship of sorts, insofar as Scossi had any friendships or knew how to maintain them. At the time, following Scossi up the steps to her flat at the back of the house, both women laden with armfuls of spare ribs, Martha had no idea that she was only the second person who had been invited in 'for a cuppa', in the last five years....she tried not to look too horrified or to turn up or hold her nose, as she walked down the hallway, filled on either side with floor to ceiling stacks of old magazines and papers.

"the Spare Ribs are in the bathroom, but we'll leave em here for now" said Scossi, plonking her armful on top of a pile of newspapers at the end of the kitchen table

FLOODING IN THE SOUTHWEST/WE'VE HAD A LOT OF WEATHER ROUND HERE/AT NIGHT I HEAR the trees creaking in the park like ancient wardrobe doors held on rusty hinges/ last night the moaning of the trees in the wind woke me up in its cacophony/

]
]
]
[ ]

]

ME AND MY STICK – LOW TECH BUT HIGH RISK AND HIGH VULNERABILITY IN THESE BUSY CITY STREETS/students don't see me – I am not visible with a stick/I raise the stick above my head – then the traffic sees me/ in the chair zooming along I am high tech and low vulnerability/ in the chair I am moving at their pace – this people seem to be able to cope with – they smile at me in my chair/in my chair I appear to be their kind of crip – getting on with my life/the pace of my walking with the stick is too slow for them – sometimes people try and walk with me, but most give up/ with...

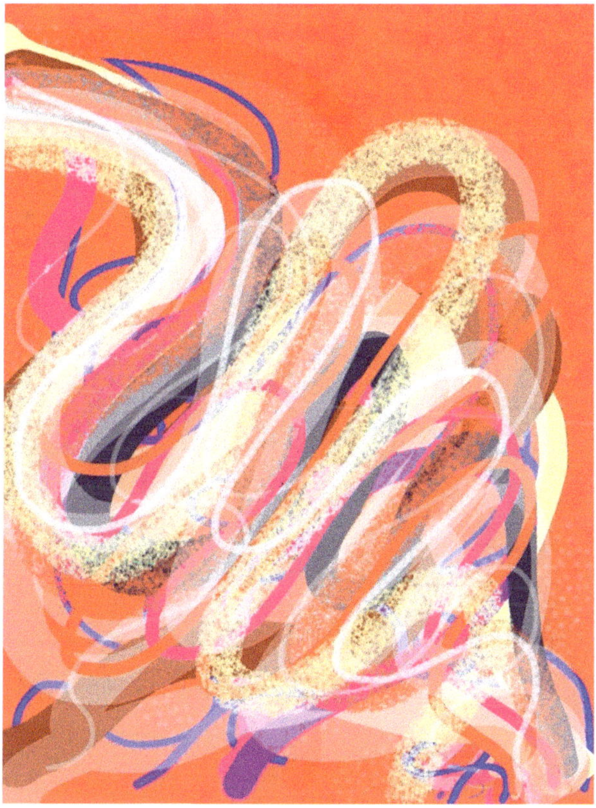

fox tracks in the snow

Fourth plateau

Early morning silence/ docx

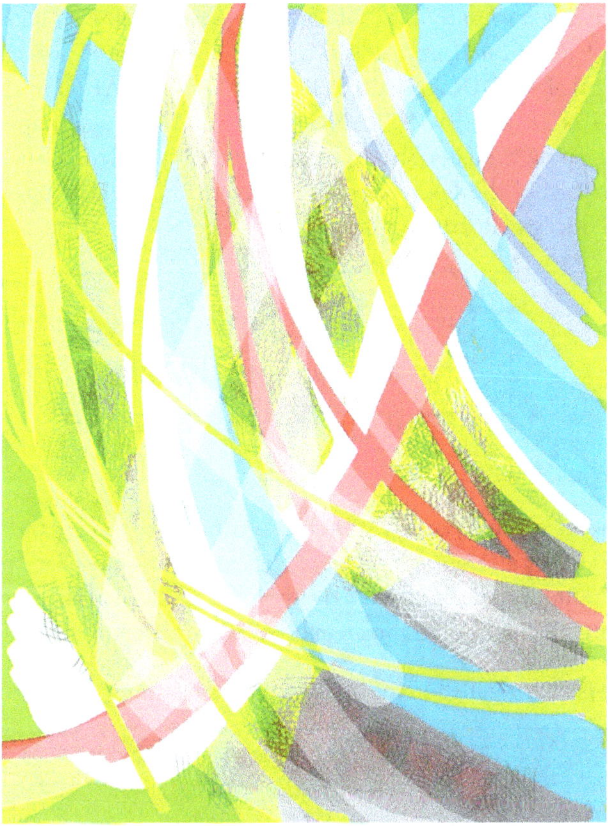

residual traces in the grass 2

Starring at the Park: A Poetic Autoethnographic Inquiry, Jane Speedy, 117–137.

EARLY MORNING SILENCE/THE SILVER LAPTOP SLID AWAY FROM HER LAP, AND PLUMMETED ONTO THE CARPET/A DULL THUD SOMEWHERE/SHE COULDN'T TELL WHETHER *it was inside or outside her head/she could not get off the floor and her left arm was all wonky/ slow motion manoevres/she made several attempts to lift the laptop up from under her, until she finally got hold of it with her right hand and threw it up onto the bed/ Her body collapsed completely onto the carpet/ [she had definitely fallen out of bed – an extraordinary event – and now she REALLY could not get up off the floor] she floundered around for a few minutes, wriggling her right leg and arm/ a broken windmill/ she made no progress/ she tried to call the others, but her voice came out in a whisper/ she could hear them moving around in the house downstairs, but they could not hear her/ she just stayed where she was and stared at the carpet/***AN AMBULANCE TO THE BRI**/DOG BARKING/ DOORBELL RINGING/VOICES:/STRANGE VOICES/clanking equipment/metal on metal/up off the floor/strong arms/into a canvas chair/clomping down the stairs/leaving the house/clanking through the night/sirens wailing/down the Gloucester Road/we stop/

> Bristol Royal Infirmary/
> Ambulances only/ No
> Parking/ Tow away zone

People in green pyjamas, stretcher/ gurney/bed/ Grey and white striped nurses (They all have names out of Dickens novels like Clara and Grace/) At some point she wakes on ward twelve wearing green pyjamas, surrounded by beds filled with elderly women in brushed bri-nylon nighties/

There is a torn leaflet on the bedside table declaring:

> 'Strokes are the biggest cause of disability in the developed world and the number three killer of adults in the UK (after heart disease and cancer)'/

She is not dead/she is awake in ward twelve, fussed over by Grace and Clara in grey and white and sister Chris in navy blue, alongside a herbaceous border of flower girls; all in their nighties and their eighties: lily, daisy, ivy and iris (there are two irises in fact), all flower girls except Edith from Clevedon, Sister Dorcas in the private room (private because she has MRSA and not because she's a nun we are informed) and her/

GOING TO THE GENERAL

TO THE LIFTS ON A GURNEY, SINGING 'AMY WINEHOUSE' WITH THE PARAMEDICS:

> ***'They tried to make me go to rehab/I said no! no! no! I ain't got the time…and if My Daddy thinks I'm fine… they tried to make me go to rehab, I won't go, go go!!***
>
> **(Winehouse, 2006)**

Through the tunnel under the road

out into the cobbled yard behind the old building/

this is near the bus station/

Bristol looks very different moving horizontally at speed/

the paramedics are all called Jane, how confusing/
We are going 'down the General, innit',
But I don't know the General/
The BRI I pass on the way to work every day, the General I have never even heard of/what goes on there?
None of my friends have ever had babies or hysterectomies or breast cancer or heart attacks in there, which is all we ever seem to go into hospitals to do/ I look up and I think we are going past the Arnolfini…/but when I ask, neither of the other Janes replies/now we are going past the flats at the back of St Mary Redcliffe – 'the fairest, goodliest and most famous parish church in all England', according to Elizabeth 1st – driving over cobbled backstreets/ we are arriving, going through big iron gates into the yard, the Janes are talking to night porters/this looks like the poorhouse/ more beige corridors and lifts/we are somewhere down by the floating harbour but I don't know where I am/I don't know where this is…

We are in another lift/we go through double doors and enter into a big space/we stop/I am moved onto a bed opposite the nurse's station/there are two nurses....brown stripes this time...Karen and Laura... we are out of the Dicken's books then, Karen and Laura strikes me as much more Joanna Trollope, or maybe Dan Brown/I am definitely in a book, or maybe the film of a book, or in a hospital series off the telly: more 'Holby City' than 'Casualty' I decide, although the beginning sequence of 'Casualty' was filmed here, Karen tells me later.../

'Where am I, Where am I? I don't know where I am/are my parents downstairs? I don't know where I am/'
Another patient, yet another Ivy in her nineties and in her nightie, is wailing at top pitch from the bed opposite/
'You're in hospital Ivy/you had a stroke/this is the Stroke rehab ward in the Bristol General Hospital'/

"Vascular dementia" Karen confides, thus preventing me from confessing to Ivy that I don't know where I am either and shouting out 'Where the fuck are we?' at the top of my voice/

THERE ARE OTHER BEDS IN HERE WITH PEOPLE ASLEEP/WHY DID ALL THIS HAPPEN SO LATE AT NIGHT I WONDER?
– I listen to Ivy moaning on and on, wondering where her parents are, *'are they upstairs?'*, she asks...
[It was not until three weeks later when Jane Thomas came to visit me and walked around the ward looking out of all the windows and reporting on what she saw, that I was able to orient myself to exactly where I was on my map of Bristol.... this hospital was behind the pub on the basin opposite the River Station and Monica and Mark's narrow boat.....]

– I listen to Laura and Karen discussing what they will wear to the staff Christmas party.....

and then I too am asleep....

'blanuk!'
I am woken by a bloodcurdling scream 'blanuk!'
Katerina is from Czechoslovakia, Karen explains, as she passes the end of my bed, going to comfort the woman in the bed on my left who screams out "blanuk' once again, into the night

One of the most mysterious of
semi-
speculations is
one
would suppose,
that of one
Mind's
Imagining into
Another

(Keats, cited in Carson, 2002 , p. 186)

'She understands a lot of English, but she doesn't speak it'

'blaaaanuk!'
Katerina has bright red hair, topped at the parting by an inch of white root, and is clearly much vexed about the 'blanuk' situation.

IN THE FRENCH FILM 'AMOUR' THE LEAD CHARACTER HAS A SECOND STROKE/This strips her of language and most movement, she loses a lot of power and control in her life – she can still spit her food out with her former spirit/

When one particular 'carer' comes to look after her all her husband can hear from her is 'mal, mal, mal, (hurts, hurts, hurts)' the carer tells him that this is just a reflex and she could be saying anything

like mum, mum,
mum/but she isn't,
and he listens to her
and eventually he
sacks the carer/then
they have no help/
he is old too/their
system has reached
tipping point/he
seals up the flat and
kills them both/the
film is called love/it
is shot through the
eyes of the husband/

It made me think
about what our
tipping point might
be here – of how
important it is to
have people on my
side who love me, of
how important love
is/how important is
it to us to be clever
cripples, to be seen
as clever? I delight
in telling people I
am a professor and
seeing their eyes
widen/when I gained
consciousness in hos-
pital the first thing I
asked for was poetry
– I wanted to see if I
could still read and
understand it/was I
still clever? language
would be a terrible,

unimaginable loss
for me/ what if I had
a second stroke? the
power visual and
textual language
gives me to make my
way and have my say
in the world would be
a terrible loss/ who
am I without lan-
guage? Would I still
be in here, trapped
without speech, a
silent language-filled
vacuum – language
is the wrong word
here, we do not know
that she did not have,
that I would not
have, my own inside
language – I am
moving on to another
French film here –
the 'diving bell and
the butterfly'(Bauby,
2008) – where the
film is shot through
the eyes, and follow-
ing the text written
by the person 'locked
in'/
communication is
the word I am look-
ing for – am I still me
without the power
to communicate?
would I still have
relationships?/
how?

This film 'amour'
(Haneke, 2012) – a
hit film, I found pro-
foundly moving and
brilliantly scripted
– there is a scene just
before tipping point
shot from inside the
husband's mind's
eye/he has a night-
mare that someone
rings the flat door-
bell/he answers the
door, but there is no-
one there… he goes
into the hallway…
the lift is all boarded
up… he walks out
into the hallway and
finds it flooded… he
is ankle deep… then
someone grabs him
from behind in the
dark and puts a hand
across his mouth,
we can hear his wife
calling him from
the flat… he wakes
up with a start…he
looks at her beside
him, and we know
in retrospect that
this was the tipping
point/but this was
his nightmare, not
hers…

I'd urge you all to go
and see this film…

Mal, mal, mal….
I never understood
before that dis-
ability hurt and
was exhausting/I
thought people in
wheelchairs were
just like me with
some bits missing –
not bits that carried
on hurting/I did not
realise how tiring it
all was or how long it
all took/

IT IS STANDARD PRACTICE FOR ACADEMICS TO DIVIDE THEIR READING / LIKE THEIR THOUGHTS/ INTO READING FOR 'THE PROJECT' AND other reading /this is rather like the compartments that hive off 'academic prose' from poetry, field notes and shopping lists but it became evident during this study that everything I was reading – in the feminist reading group, the newspaper and in the bath – was all slipping around in the mix and providing scaffolding for staring at the park. Thus Kathleen Swift's 'the Morville hours' which we were reading in the blue-stockings group became the underpinning for a way of mapping traces left by the Victorian park builders and the BBC Wales (2014) production of Under Milk Wood for the centenary of Dylan Thomas's birth led to further readings of other park ghosts/ with Mrs. Dai Bread 1 and Mrs. Dai Bread 2 in mind my staring caught traces of ancient people trudging along the coffin paths over to Baddock woods. Indeed, there were any number of contenders in the park most days for the roles of Polly Garter and No Good Boyo. Books blew in as sources by a
variety of means, mostly serendipity and a westerly wind/
I wonder about these predecessors in the park. Were they people like me, the Victorian park builders or what were the bronze age funeral goers like, what were their preoccupations?
Finkel (2014), having spent his life studying the Babylonians and Mesopotamians, in their own words, concludes that the minds of these people were equally complex and corrupt and their considerations very similar to our

own. There are, after all, only about 40 generations between our selves and Nebuchanezzar, which does not give us much time to have evolved very differently. Perhaps, in ontological as opposed to chronological versions of temporality (Hein, 2013), all peoples are present and contemporary in their emotional power and resonance? According to Hein, quoting Deleuzian concepts of Aion rather than Chronos, 'Ontological time is a time without the present, one that includes both an absolute past and an absolute future. Unlike chronological time (i.e., the time of historical unfolding), ontological time consists of a past that never took place, one that was never lived through' (p. 493).

> The horse chestnut and I were co-authoring this park and its stories. We had our preferred stories and subjugated knowledges and made alliances together to deconstruct authentic identity claims, to unpack identity claims that foreclosed on multiple discourses, we preferred winged creatures and peasant coffin trails to other more mundane and everyday practices as staree and starer.

EXPERIENCING SEVERE PALPITATIONS, THE PROFESSOR OF POETIC INQUIRY COULD NO LONGER CONTAIN HERSELF/ CONVULSED WITH RAGE, SHE LUNGED FORWARD WITH HER RIGHT WING and brought it down with great force on the back of the mayor's neck/turquoise feathers flew about in all directions/he staggered, slid on the tiles and tripped backwards over his feet into the paddling pool behind/he reared up out of the pool, belching and spluttering out feathers/ she remained balanced on the side in a squatting position/bashing him over the head again and again, each time he rose out of the water/the bruising was terrible/great red and blue/black welts appeared all over his neck, forehead, face and upper chest/ he was easy pickings for a winged professor/after about ten minutes they both seemed to tire of this game/he stopped bobbing up and drifted away, face down, into the centre of the paddling pool and she stopped clonking him with her wings but remained, crouched, watching him intently, at the side of the pool/how easy it was to kill another human being, she thought, registering that this was what she had just done/then she turned and took off, wings outstretched and flew back, circling the park triumphantly and straight through the window of her bedroom eyrie, leaving the mayor floating face down in what seemed to be a pool of feathers, just as the sun came up/

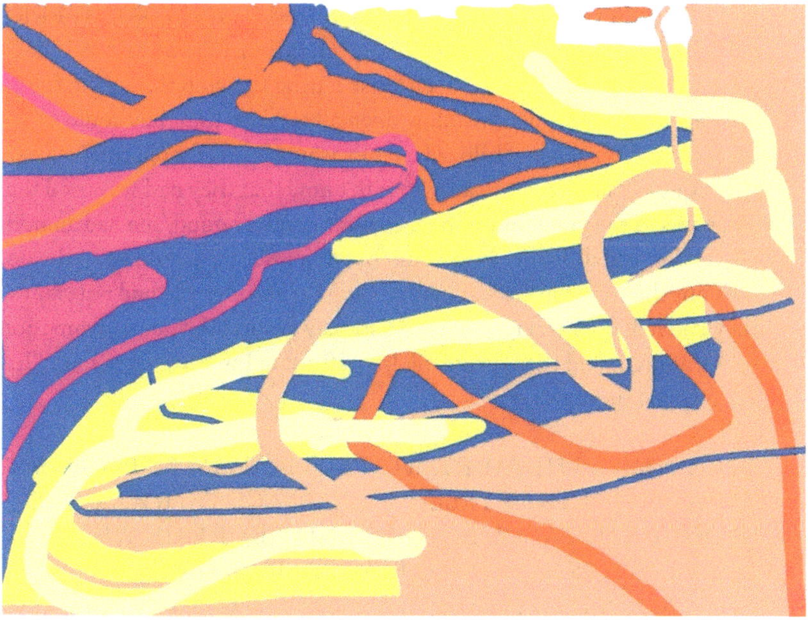

tracks through the park

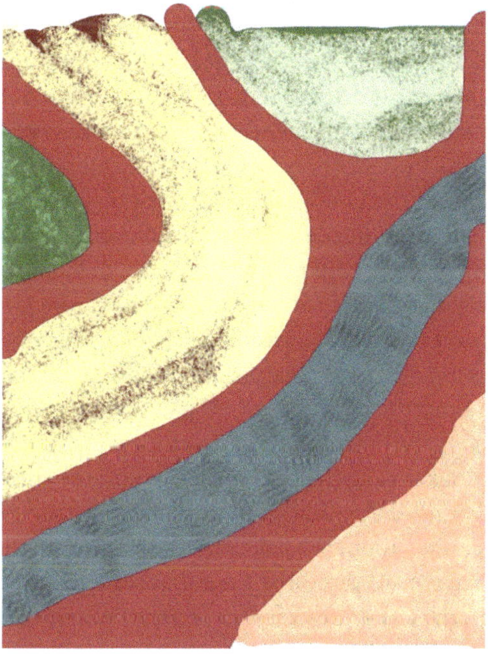

coffin trail to baddock woods

SCOSSI WAS UPSET TO THINK THAT HER GRANDAD'S FERRETS HAD DESERTED HER, AND THE HOUSE FELT EMPTY WITHOUT THEM, but she knew it had been a risk letting them off the lead in the park/ she had left the basement window open all week so that they could come back and have a game of billiards if they wanted, just for old times sake, but she thought that they probably wouldn't now that they had savoured the pleasures of the great outdoors/they were gone for good/she had an odd aching feeling and difficulty breathing/Martha said she should go to the doctor's but she thought she was just missing the ferrets/ she had not slept since they had left, but rather, wandered listlessly around the house, from room to room, at night and then dozed all day in front of the back room fire/ She had really loved those ferrets/

FOR A WHILE THE PARK IMITATED LIFE 'AS SEEN ON TV' WITH GREAT SWATHES OF YELLOW AND BLACK TAPE WRAPPED AROUND THE PADDLING POOL AND FIGURES IN WHITE ROMPER SUITS GLIMPSED BETWEEN THE HEDGES THAT SURROUNDED IT/The police didn't seem to walk anywhere any more, but rather, drove stripy cars and assorted white vans at great speed up and down Maurice road all day, only stopping beside the paddling pool entrance with great screechings of brakes/It was fascinating/
Abbi decided to complete the rest of her marking at the table in the bay window and Martha and Scossi took to 'jogging' around the park together with uncharacteristic frequency/ there were countless white vans, packed with news teams and camera crews, parked all around the perimeter for several days/living in a house overlooking the park had always held a certain cachet, but these days the phrase 'my bedroom window overlooks the park' evoked blatant prurience from all but the most virtuous of fellow citizens/ Abbi took longer and longer over each assignment, spending hours of her time staring over the top of her reading glasses at the police circus that was taking place across the road/Martha and Scossi would start at a reasonable jogging pace along the north side of the park, skirting the children's area and then whizz along the downhill strait past the toilets and slowly move uphill across the Effingham and Leopold road end until they reached the tape barriers that surrounded the paddling pool/here they would stop and walk and listen to the conversations the police were all having on their radios/it really was just like having an episode of 'the bill' recorded outside your house, an impression given all the more credence by the presence of so many journalists and photographers/

"What's this crap about feathers, they're all on about? asked Martha 'Dunno' replied Scossi, "But they all seem to be talking about feathers/hasn't been on the news has it? – oh look there's Abbi working at home again, let's go and interrupt her shall we?

YOUR LEAVES
GREEN TENDER SHOOTS
A COVERING OF SORTS
YOUR TRUNK EXPOSED AMIDST THE FROTH
AND TULLE

Your small
Delicate fruit
Begin to appear more
Expansive in the spring sunlight
Slow green

Your buds
In hiding for
Later in the cycle
Deep red and glorious absence
Held high

Hidden
Candelabras
Of deep red blossom and
new buxom greenness waiting to
Sprout forth

No such
Thing as coyness
Or authenticity
In your arboreal lexicon:
treeness

Innate
Green/Grey Treeness
Is all the contribution
You are required to make in life
On earth

Standing
Weeping bare-trunked
Cankerous tears for all
To see and stare at in the park
You dare

Neighbour
You have stood there
Sobbing down your trunk in
Front of my bay window/your forked
Branches sodden

With sap
Moulding canker
Pouring out unabashed
You stand and stare through my window
Alone

You've lived
Alongside my
Busy little life spent
Ignoring you and your plight. You
Watch me

Just as
I do not see
You standing and weeping
Beside me in the park for years
And years

Watching
Horse chestnuts grow
Has been an unusual
Year-long occupation and not
So strange

As I
Might have thought it
At one time. Idling and staring
Have brought new mores to
The fore

I see
And read about
Your canker now, diseased,
Like most of your kind who dwell in
England

WALKING/

THEY DEFINITELY LIKE WALKING/ALL THESE EFFORTS TO GET ME WALKING/walking with a helper/walking with a zimmer/ walking with a stick/walking *independently*/the world of rehab is obsessed with walking/perpendicularity/getting up on our hind legs/it's a very precarious business/as I look out of my bedroom window at the park every morning, I can't help feeling that the dogs have got it sussed/none of this precarious perpendicular pitching forwards for them – a limb at each corner, squarely put – and one paw placed securely in front of another/just a short walk/how far can you walk?/can you walk to my car? /how far can you walk on your own?/20 metres is the crucial distance – there's money in 20 metres of perpendicularity with no discomfort/ there has been no such obsession with my arm, which is equally weak since the stroke/no 'how long can you grip/hold on/ stroke the dog for' scales – all of which are equally, if not more, important to my quality of life/only legs count/for legs make you mobile – and despite the fact that there are all kinds of sticks and props and wheels to get a girl around without legs /independent legs count for more than independent arms in this business/nobody really cares if you can get your bra or your socks on, but they mind a lot if you can haul yourself up onto your hind legs and strut about/George Orwell (1945) nailed it with 'four legs good: two legs better' there's something quintessentially, definingly human about perpendicularity/ Precarious living Judith Butler (2004, pp. 1–10) called it – although I don't think perpendicularity was quite what she meant, when she spoke of taking 'collective responsibility to reap what we have sown'/ in her book "precarious life' /Butler took the 9/11 terrorist attacks on the USA as the vantage point from which to view life's precariousness and examine and critique the ensuing privatised and depoliticised acts of grief and mourning/ if I take my stroke as the vantage point from which to view life's precariousness and this immense will to perpendicularity (mine and others) as some kind of individualised and depoliticised tramway riding roughshod over grief and mourning for the loss of an arm.... But surely this is craziness, we all want to walk, don't we? /don't we? /for there is a politics to limb loss – all limbs being equal, some it seems are more equal than others in the eyes of the NHS and society generally/paralysed limbs too, it would seem, are worth more than no limbs/ when I asked about the medics chopping my arm off and getting me a false electronic one, I was dismissed as 'weird'/ Was this weird? I don't know/ I would far rather have my own working hand than this floppy thing hanging down from my shoulder, but why not get a digitally operated new one?/ What's the difference between that and a wheelchair?/ social convention and the social desirability of ambulant activity/ Kate at hydrotherapy tells me that a robotic arm connects with and uses the existing neurological pathways so a new robotic arm won't assist where there has been neurological damage, only physiological damage/ Damn/I really fancied a new turquoise arm/ have you seen that film: Avatar?/

But this year is different

]
]
]
]

[ ]

]
]
]
]

[ ]

/December 28th/ an incident/ a noise in the night/the oak tree next to the horse chestnut is down/ ripped at the fork of her trunk, her longest and heaviest branch has fallen into the park/ no-one is hurt/ bald-headed men come and look at the damage/ neighbourhood conversations take place/I watch different groups of people come and stand around the fallen tree/all day people come with hacksaws and chain saws to glean pieces and branches for their fireplaces/by nightfall the fallen treetop is bare /January 3rd/when we come back from Wales the stripped-bare tree is lying in pieces in the park/ people pass by and try and pick up the logs/ but they are too big for them to carry/ everything that can be taken home already has been/these great logs are waiting for the park keepers to clear them/my horse chestnut looks on/ still bleeding furiously from the middle/wondering what her faithful companion has done to garner all this human attention/no-one notices her weeping/ it is getting very cold and her twigs and branches are covered in a film of frost every morning/not only am I alongside the Horse Chestnut/watching and waiting and idling and staring/but she is also alongside me / so vibrantly and materially and obviously alongside that it is difficult to ascertain exactly who had ignored whom for the past thirteen years of games with absence and presence /aspects were definitely and reciprocally turned to each other/the staring felt mutual/ although quite who was starer and who was staree was difficult to ascertain/

not only was I alongside the horse chestnut, watching and waiting and idling and staring, but the horse chestnut was also alongside me – so vibrantly and materially and obviously alongside that it was difficult to ascertain exactly who had ignored who for the past thirteen years – aspects were definitely and reciprocally turned to each other, and the staring felt mutual, although quite who was starer and who was staree was difficult to ascertain.

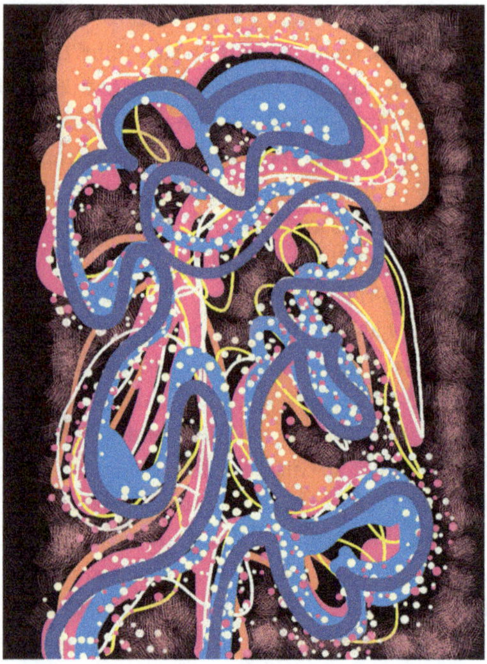

non-human
tracks

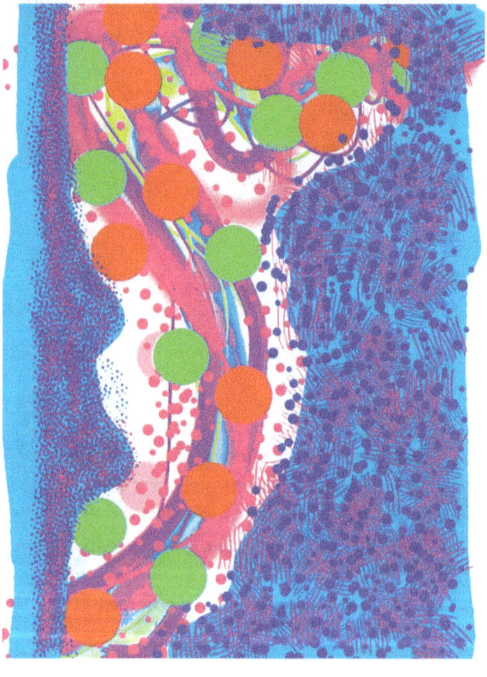

more non-human
tracks

Plane blight/oak decline/beech and hornbeam wilt/horse chestnut bleeding canker/ash die back and elm disease/a human lifetime's stretch of damage/ The trees are dying/ slowly dying as they grow/One thousand years up and quickly down/bleeding darkly from the middle/ rotten sap seeping out/

THERE IS WRITING AND THEN THERE IS PAINTING/BOTH REQUIRE THE IPAD, A HAND, A LAP, A VIEW OF THE PARK/Both are processes of looking at the park and setting down what is there on the screen, but they are different practices/ The writing forms itself somewhere in my body/brain/I can hear the writing and I can hear the process of it forming/ I hear the words as they form on the screen in front of me/sometimes I get a sore throat from not saying the words I am forming in writing/even though they are set down differently from my practices of speaking/ the writing is linear, a series of lines, one after the other, one under the other/set down in an ordered way/in black on white or sepia on cream or blue on yellow, in any case in dark on light/
the painting does not form itself inside me before I get sight of the park/I have written about the writing first, but in fact, when I was in hospital it was the drawing that came first/sketchbooks and pastels came before pens and lined paper/I don't know how this work becomes writing or painting/ it is the same process of going over to sit by the window with the iPad/ the same kind of looking out/and I know, just know, if I am going to write or paint/ sometimes my mind is full of words that burst out onto the page/sometimes the writing has been piecing itself together in my mind before I get to the window/and I have to get these out before sight of the park overwhelms with the need for painting/ for setting out the structure and texture and colour beneath the surface/then I am filled with purpose/moments of flow or what Virginia Woolf (2002) called 'moments of being' in relation to what I see and hear in the park/in these moments the park is not something I observe or participate in/nor something greatly other/but both the park and I/like the horsechestnut and I /are in the same moment/being together/we are not 'othering' each other, not caught up in the treeness of trees or the womanliness of women/ but more than adjacency is happening here /we are a moment of 'just-thisness' in the Deleuzian sense (Davies & Gannon, 2013) / there is a

shrinking and at the same time an expanding into oneness, in the moment of being in the space between us/ we are no longer staree or starer the one with the other, but rather, elements in a mutual staring event/ Klee (1920) says 'art does not reproduce the visible: rather, it makes visible' and in this making visible through finger painting the fruits/objects of my practices of staring, I am making visible the abstractions of colour and substance and shape that can be traced just beneath the park in the view from my window, in an attempt, to quote Klee, again, to 'reveal the reality that is behind visible things, thus expressing the belief that the visible world is merely an isolated case in relation to the universe and that there are many more other, latent realities' (p. 79)/ Indeed, just beneath the visible lurk the residual traces of other former, older spaces: the site of the wellington bomber crash in world war two, or even the farm owned by Mr. Derham, the bootmaker, that existed here before the park was laid out in 1895 in order to provide a green space for the local people, who were living in the 'third most congested' city in England (after London and Manchester) clogged with the wastes of myriad surrounding factories (friendsofstandrewspark.ning.com/) There are times when I sit here and the park seems full of futures and histories and images/vestiges of other semi-visible patterns under the veil of the 'now'/ The park is brimming with palimpsests, with the presence of absences/it is as if there were, as Virginia Woolf (2002, p. 85) put it 'some real thing behind appearances. I make it real by putting it into words. It is only by putting it into words that I make it whole'/Unlike Virginia, my words still get somewhat in the way of making the absent present, but not so the images I make/ the images seem to be able to penetrate the layers between me and the stream I am swimming in/

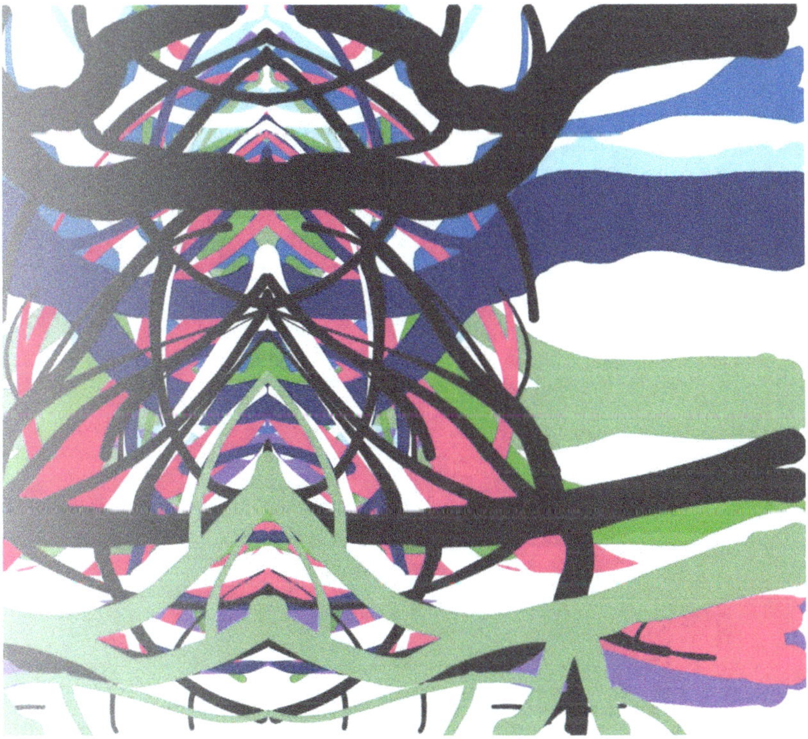

night branches

Fifth plateau

Park haiku/winged/docx

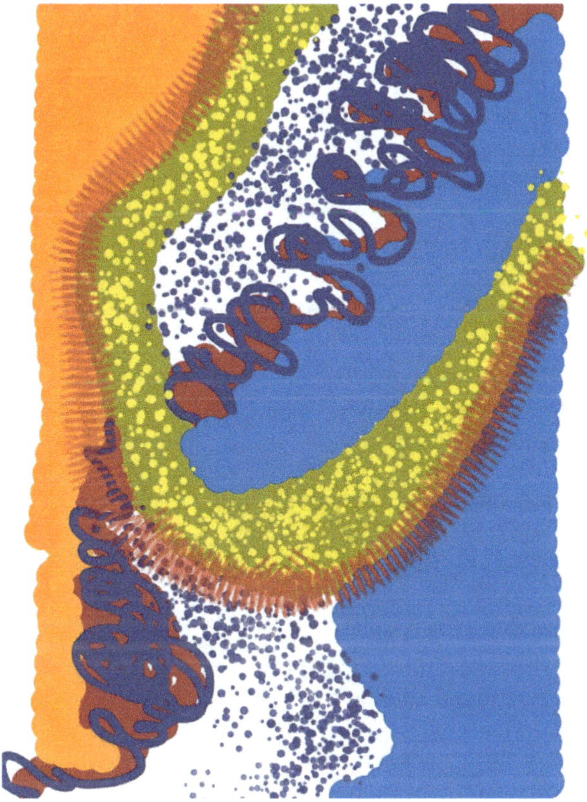

night flight

Starring at the Park: A Poetic Autoethnographic Inquiry, Jane Speedy, 139–157.

PARK HAIKU/
A FOX LOITERS BY
THE AVENUE OF PLANE TREES/
AS I DRAW THE BLINDS

New grass is growing/
human patterns linger on
ready-made pathways

The dawn chorus stops/
Starling and seagull gangs plough
up old dog dung

the park day starts with
the dogs/unless you include
The gentle man in

his torn yellow coat/
with his long-handled
grabber/ to scoop up litter

whose anger simmers/
as he dragss his black bin bag
around behind him

dogs chase squirrels up
trees/leaving scents for trackers
and foxy sniffers

my favourite couple
with the German Shepherd/
stroll round holding hands

this fine couple in
hats /walk the perimeter
twice – sometimes three times

the maths lecturer
Often meets her at the gate
with his retriever

He lollops with an
academic optimism
in a tarnished world

Tikh Nhat Han does
walking meditations with
a similar lollop/

she calls her poodle
'Heinrich the dog' and solves no
equations walking/

dogs and their walkers
share their morning moment with
lycra-clad joggers

and Bert /Running round
in his tea-shirt and baggy
old shorts/red in the face

in contrast with the
old bloke serenely doing
Tai Chi by the wall

Then come the children
criss-crossing the park to school/
on bikes and scooters

small ones with parents/
others with kitbags and books
and rucksacks and 'stuff'

cool kids bring nothing/
they swagger in late/in a group/
kicking up litter

which the wind blows side-
ways up against the hedges/
tangled and lonely/

the park suddenly
empties /the sun moves west as
starling flocks return

up goes the café/
chairs /tables /plastic cloths and
attendant seagulls

freshly baked brownies/
and people at the counter
qeueing for lattes

from strong paper cups
that blow /turning somersaults
across the wet grass

a mid morning calm
straddles the park / in a glut
of birdsong and breeze

that goes unnoticed
by the rest of the city/
then hullaballoo

bursts out of the play
park /seeing off gulls and crows/
women with buggies/

toddlers and babies
occupy the café seats/
a threatening throng/

the circus school sets
up tight ropes between the trees/
they juggle in groups

nomadic young men
practice the bongos alone/
near the dealer's bench

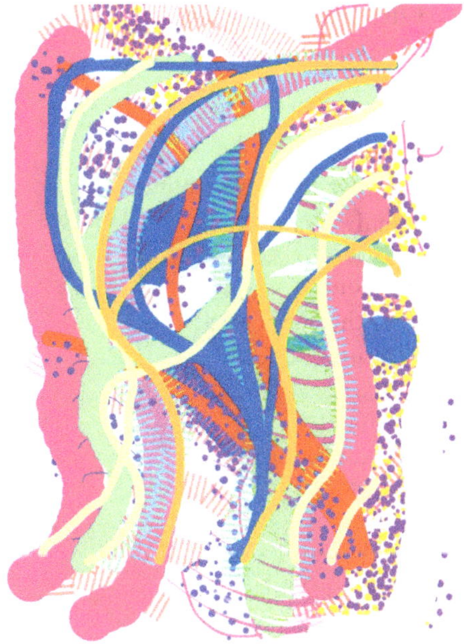

trails

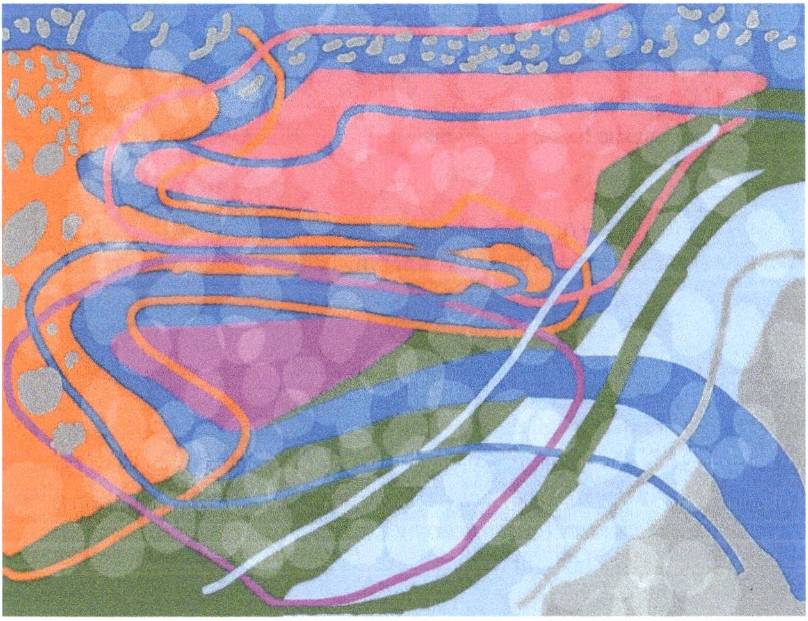

window on the park

all day battered cars
come and go on our corner
and agitated

people jerk along
the path to score some more blow/
before night draws in/

in the afternoons
students and the out of work
picnic on the grass

and play their music
too loud to hear the sparrows
chattering away/

after school the kids
corner and the café fill
with strident sounds

ice cream vendors come
and park down Somerville road
just at the top gate

games of footie start
on the flatter grassy bits/
jumpers for goal posts

people coming back
from work with their shopping bags
meander slowly home

snogging couples come
and monopolise benches
under the plane trees

they watch the café
pack away for the evening
as the daylight fades

the community
police come on foot by day
and by car at night

ignoring dealers
and punters and bench gropers
alike/some have horses

which causes a bit
of a rumpus in the caff
as they sashay through

and as the night falls
snogging turns to fucking and
dog tracks to foxes

their howling sounds wild
and desperately lonely
like the owl screeching

out to its neighbours
in the avenue of trees/
the whispering bats

and when great swathes of
birds erupt in a bold and
vertical tunnel of sound

it all begins afresh/
sometimes the cackling magpies and
creaking trees out-shine

and diminish the
supremacy of humans/
as stormy weather

sweeps in from the west
and great branches crash aground/
bringing chaos up

close to city lives
measured and controlled by men
and not by nature

this daily cycle
of parklife rituals has gone on
for a century

and more/ paths across
the park hold memories of
previous cycles

the park is like an
amphor – a jar full of memories
of people and birds

and animals that
inhabited the hedges/
left marks and made tracks

and the planting and
pruning and felling of the trees/
that stand unnoticed

their majesty out
lasting us all with our schemes
to outlast our selves

DRAWING THE PARK somehow brought her closer to the trees and its other inhabitants/ the act of drawing, being not only a drawing on but a drawing out/a curiosity about/ and an engagement with the gorgeousness and squalor of the everyday/ the pictures do not re-present the park to you any more than the writing does/but rather capture something of her process of dis(un)covery in relating newly to the trees next door as neighbours, to the horse chestnut in particular as friend and fellow invalid, and not as backdrop to her more

> An engagement with the gorgeousness and squalor of the everyday

> Families came out. They saw open sky families came out, they saw open sky for the first time in ages.
>
> We found ourselves in the first chapter of a very gripping story.
>
> (Transtroemer, 2011, p. 70)

(central) human life/ she saw how people walked and talked differently in the park/ this five acre in-between-country-and-city space in the midst of the city streets/the park was at the same time more relaxed and faster paced than the surrounding streets/she wanted to convey something of the sadness of the trees/her tree/ in her images where their sadness meets a sadness in us that/in its Christ-like recognition and empathic greeting/somehow lessens the sadness in us all/her recent brush with death gave her no greater insights/ the horse chestnut/the other side of her window/ hiding her canker from public gaze/met us halfway/rendered us collaborators in life/

WHY HAD THE GODS NOT COMPENSATED HER SUFFICIENTLY FOR HER LOSS? /this weakness down her left side had not brought any special compensatory gifts as such losses and signs of weakness did in Greek myths/she had not yet been transformed into a seer or sage, and even the performance of her newly minted role of the 'happy cripple' felt like such an effort/she had lost her left side/what did she get in exchange? / it was a well-known fact that blind people were all able to tune pianos and deaf people had amazing peripheral vision and second sight/what did broken people with black holes in their brains where thoughts used to be, get in exchange?/ the god Hermes had winged feet and was the Usain Bolt of his day/bet he was a staree and a half when he whizzed round the park for his early morning jog/that Rosemarie Garland-Thomson (2009) would have had a field day with Hermes/'He was my kind of hybrid-staree, that Hermes', she would have said if they'd have met /staring bespeaks involvement, and being stared at demands a response/a staring encounter is a dynamic struggle – starers enquire, starees lock eyes or flee, and starers advance or retreat; one moves forward and the other moves back/ (p. 3)

Now me, I've always fancied a pair of wings/not on my feet/ proper muscular wings/ fell down again last Sunday night in the sitting room/I was trying to move the books and stuff that had accumulated on the table by my side/people, well-intentioned, bring it all to me when they come crip-visiting and leave it on the table where it accumulates/ poems; books about imagined lives; packets of flower seeds; bath salts; packets of oil pastels; chocolates; a paisley painted trowel – in short, everything a poorly girl could need/they send them through the post or just put them down beside me when they sit down to 'visit' and never see the effects of all this accumulation of 'stuff'/
'I couldn't come empty-handed' they say/ 'why not I go everywhere one-handed'/I think/but somehow that bubble never appears above my head/that would be rude and ungrateful and wouldn't do/
Anyway, I was having a go at moving all the stuff, which was quite heavy, actually, when I overbalanced, bounced my head and back down the wall and landed on my bum, legs tucked awkwardly backwards underneath me in the sitting room/could have been worse, as Simon, the paramedic, said on the blue report forms he had to fill in/there was a green report form too for me (or my carer) to fill out at our leisure and yellow copies of everything for everybody/anyway, I don't know whether it was the bump that did it, but there was a real soreness starting in my shoulders/an underskin lumpiness started erupting, followed by a hollow, whimsical inner creaking sound a bit like the out-puffs of an old harmonium, and I knew instantly that my much longed-for wings were at last growing/I could feel the tingling of the soft top feathers finally sprouting just below the skin/'this'll really give 'em something to stare at in the park', I thought.

I knew instantly that my much longed-for wings were at last growing

all the next day there was a tingling and separating of skin, bone and feather all down my back and legs/I had to sit a long way forward on my chair, almost on the edge/by last

Tuesday lunchtime I couldn't contain my excitement and hobbled upstairs to the back bedroom to have a look in the full-length mirror at my newly developing expanse of wing/I was hoping for black crow-like feathers, but these were even better in a bright shimmering peacock-blue and green with gold-rimmed purple peacock's eyes below the shoulder joint/wow! here was my compensation/I had at last become a winged creature, like Hermes, talk of the park/

the Greek god Hephaestus, son of Hera and Zeus, king and queen of heaven, was thrown down from Olympus to earth by his warring parents, with the result that he was crippled and walked with a limp/when he grew up, he was rewarded by the gods with marriage to Aphrodite, goddess of love (Ebenstein, 2006)/I would rather have wings/
that night I tried them out, tentatively opening the bedroom window, and casting all my usual thoughts and fears of vertigo asunder, I jumped straight out to fly across the park/I had finally been compensated for my left side weakness by the gods, but at the same time, become filled, like Hephaestus, with a vengeful anger/
swooping down amongst the trees, the park was silent and still/the noise of traffic on the M32 seemed to fade into the distance and from above it seemed that the trees in the park all stood in a state of hushed reverie, as if they were waiting for something to happen/ the avenue of horse chestnuts in the middle of the park was home to a colony of whispering bats, who flocked out to join me as I swooped over the café/

By the end of the following week I had become quite used to my wings/there was quite an art to getting them in under my clothes, which made getting dressed in the mornings take even longer than it usually did/I tried to ignore the fact that on the ground the wings added to the asymmetry of my broken, unruly body/with the left wing dragging along behind me on the carpet like my leg/once launched from the window sill, however, the wings came into their own, each wing beating against the air with an ease that the rest of my body had lost/by day I lived with my gifts covered over/I had no desire to become known for my circus-show freakery/ but how I longed for those cool summer nights; for the feeling of speed as I swished high above the trees/I stayed out regularly night after night, only returning home as the dawn light began to creep up and glance off the shimmer of my wings/every night I slid back over the window sill, wing muscles creaking and groaning with the effort of folding themselves up under my shoulder blades once again/the park was my playground/I was its creature/FUCK HERMES/

> I lived with my gifts covered over/I had no desire to become known for my circus show freakery

> The ethical question of politics, or of responsibility has always haunted me, as I imagine it haunts all the fireflies irresistibly attracted by the flame of the art-candle.
>
> (Cixous & Calle-Gruber, 1997, p. 6)

INSIDER/OUTSIDER
TALKING ABOUT SUICIDE AS POWER AND CONTROL
TAKES AWAY PROFESSIONAL RESPONSES
takes away protocols and knowing what to do and leaves us
there together as two human beings making sense of stuff
together

which reminds me
of the nights in the park outside my house
a few weeks ago, when after and before and during
the so called 'Bristol riots'
I hung out chatting to
the boys – and they were all boys – in hoodies
all hanging out and chatting and drinking and smoking in the park

I was there being/becoming someone's mum on the way back from the co-op
which was okayish and we got chatting
and then the next night walking the dog, chatting because

we'd chatted before and then the next night because stroking dogs
is okay /quite cool a thing you can do in a hood...

and then one of them recognised me
from the project at the university, I'd talked to him before
and then suddenly I wasn't a mum or a dog walker or a silly old git
suddenly I was a fucking professor
which may have blown it, because the next night and the next night they were not there any more....

Am I writing rubbish? Attending to aesthetics, not ethics and will the sisters swoop down like Nussbaum on Butler (Nussbaum, 1999)[1] and question the connection of this writing to 'the real situation of real women'? I tenderly write towards Mabel and Ivy and believe they will consume such a text fragment by fragment and like archaeologists will dust off each scrap and hold it up to the light, but what if they, like Lather and Smithies' angels[2], would have preferred a supermarket book? Is this a betrayal?

TWO GROUPS THAT DON'T SHARE THE PARK SPACE WELL ARE THE YUMMY MUMMIES AND THE BATS/there are large groups of brown long-eared or 'whispering' bats living in the park, mostly roosting in tree holes near the centre or in the eaves of the church on Maurice Road by day and coming out to feed at night/ the yummy mummies are rarely in the park after lunch, never mind after dark, but on the occasions when something or someone has disturbed the bats in their tree holes in the centre of the park by the café in the morning (usually by throwing sticks and balls up into the tree canopies when the bats are sleeping) the bats come out during the day and flutter quite low to the ground, usually at designer buggy level/...

IT WAS A KANTHA SHAWL MADE FROM TWO OLD SARIS STITCHED TOGETHER WITH GREEN AND ORANGE THREAD/ one side was plain forest green silk cloth and the other a richly patterned peacock-feather paisley pattern in gold, turquoise, orange and viridian green/like all already-worn clothing/each side of her shawl carried with it the spectral traces of its own history/each side of the garment contained fragments from the lives and memories of previous owners that remained folded into its fabric/her daily unfolding of the shawl witnessed an uncovering of these forgotten memories and soon her bedroom floor was strewn with the post-colonial secrets, lies and memories of other lives on other continents/ after a couple of years of owning the shawl the corners of her room had filled up with the dust, silt and sediment of other people's lives and landscapes/the shawl and its stories were calling her to Jodhpur/she became consumed with the need to trace the fragments of stories that she had overheard whispered in the corners of her bedroom back to the place that they had come from/she was also losing weight quite dramatically during this time, a phenomenon that other people had started to notice/ people who knew her closely began begging her not to wear her shawl any more/friends urged her to buy a different shawl/one made from newly

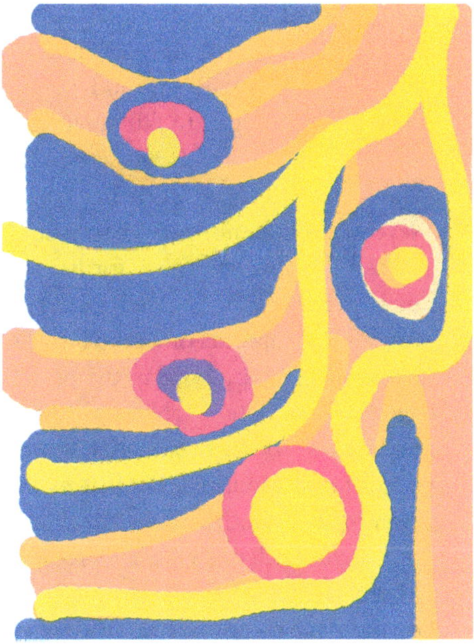

kantha shawl

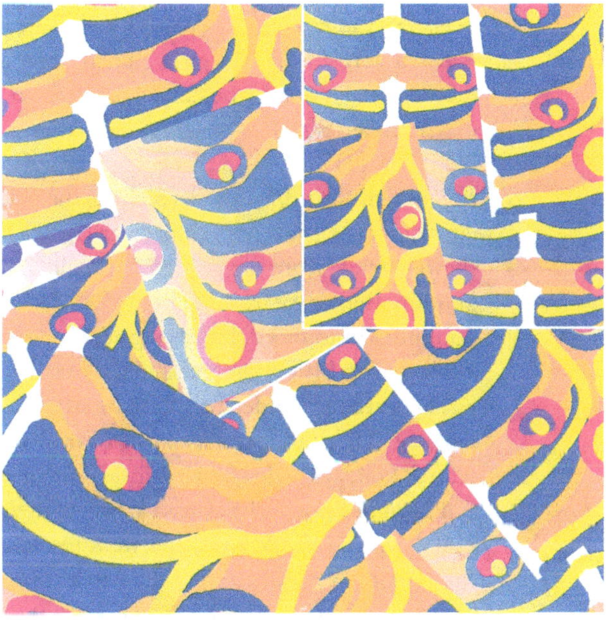

multiple kantha shawls

woven, fresh, unstoried cloth, but the professor just wrapped the Kantha shawl more tightly and determinedly around her shoulders/ then her hair began to fall out/every morning when she woke her pillow was covered in great clumps of thick grey curly hair/she consulted several doctors, none of whom could find any discernible medical cause for her sudden loss of hair and body weight /finally pronouncing them symptoms of work-related stress and prescribing a long holiday/the professor managed to negotiate a sabbatical term from her University, which meant that she could have a full three months away just as long as she crammed her entire annual workload into the rest of the academic year/she promptly booked a flight to India/
on the plane she found herself sat next to a lovely, smiling Rajasthani girl who shrieked with delight as she flung the shawl over her shoulders, revealing its peacock paisley underside:
'Oh I'm sorry', said the girl. 'But my grandmother used to have a beautiful sari made out of that material'/
'Well it might have been this very piece of fabric', replied the professor, smoothing the paisley side of the shawl out across her lap/ 'This shawl is made from old saris. Where did your grandmother come from?
'Jodhpur', announced the girl proudly/
'She owned a little guesthouse in the old town, just beneath the Golden temple in Mehrangarh Fortress. We used to stay with her for all the school holidays, when I was little, and help run her guesthouse/I never saw her wear the peacock sari, I think it was her wedding sari/ she kept it in a cedar chest in the corner of her bedroom, along with all her best saris, but she would occasionally take it out and run her

hands down the fabric, just like you are doing now and she would look at it and weep over it'/
"Yes it does make you feel sad, this side of the shawl. It makes me weep too" Agreed the professor/
'Well, I'm heading for Jodhpur old town on my sabbatical/I'm already booked in to the Hotel Raas/but perhaps I could drop in on your grandmother in her guesthouse and show her my shawl' offered the professor/
'oh no, grandma died three years ago' said the girl/
'they've made her guest house into the tourist information centre though/ so you can go and see where she lived if you like'/
they chatted on amiably for an hour or so about their families and about the role of grandmothers in particular, in holding together and keeping up family stories/then they both collapsed into a companionable silence until the plane began its descent into Jodhpur airport/ Just as she was preparing to get off the plane the professor turned to her young companion and inquired:
'your grandmother, how did she die?'
'well she was really very old, and also she was diagnosed with cancer ' said the girl/
'It was so sad visiting her when she was dying/ She took a long time to die/ ....She'd had such long, thick, black hair all her life/Her hair had been her pride and joy, but in the end, what with the chemotherapy, it all fell out..../She used to tie a scarf tightly around her head, a bit like the way you're wearing yours/I thought it looked really nice, but she never got over it, and you know what?/her hair never ever grew back like they said it would/they pronounced the cause of her death as cancer of the liver, but I reckon it was outliving her own hair that finally killed her'/

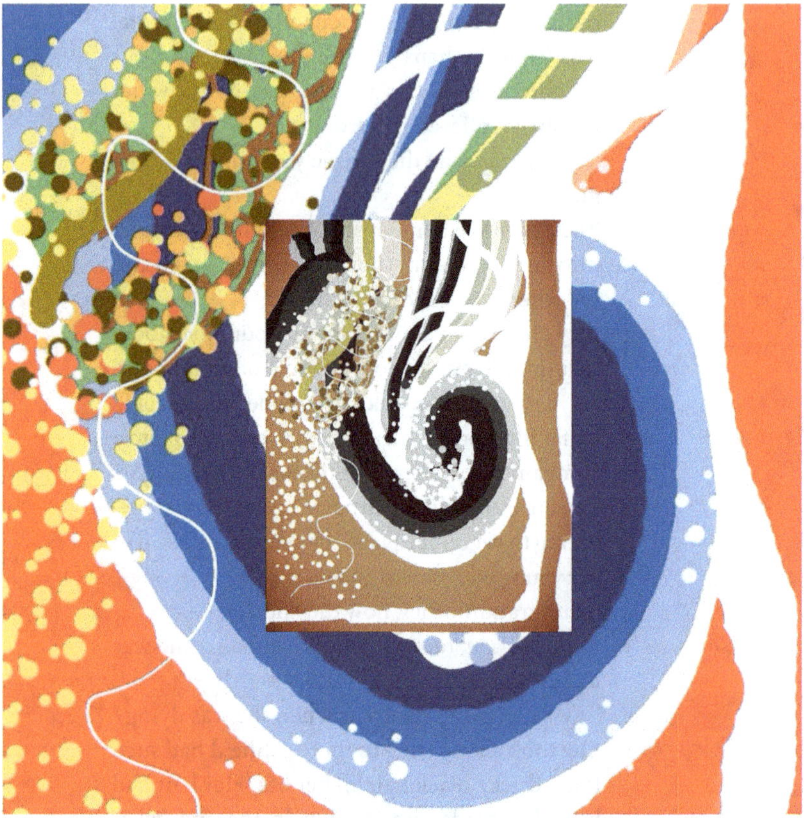

the winged creature's cloak

LYING JUST BELOW THE PARK
SURFACE/ FLOAT THE WORD
nuggets waiting for distillation/ salient sounds stick in
auditory filters/and get caught up in the text-net/
a fine-meshed sound-sieve, sharp eyes and good hearing these are all the paraphernalia needed for collecting poetic everyday comments in and around the hospital or neighbourhood/ prose is (apparently) okay for academics/ too many words put down where haiku would do?/ poems found lying on the ground/ and trodden into lino corridors/are allowed if we can trace their origins in our sacred data/our holy transcripts/this ritualised cleansing into text of that which is 'empirically' found/ according to Lahman and Richard (2014), citing the sainted Richardson (1993, 2000):

'Lousy poetry
masquerades
as research
and vice versa'

yet this whole murder inquiry/ ethnography/ life-story malarkey is nothing but a performance/ masquerade/ show me the text that masquerades as nothing and I'll give you back thin air /or the instructions for setting the timer on your boiler and the shopping list he dropped on the landing/ (he forgot the toothpaste) / these scraps could enter the holy transcripts yet as 'field notes?' / 'landing notes?'/ 'selected pages collected in the researcher's journal?'/ 'filtered /annotated litter?'/ I like the sound of 'vice-versa' (above) / lousy poetry or lousy practices of inquiry? /

I am very attuned, these days, to my body/myself in a state of becoming/ always becoming never there/being/becoming lousy/everything changing/ I am with Gale (2014, p. 1), who finds this a space or domain of 'implication and inference, suggestion and nuance, sense and intuition' I recall the word embodiment as if it was imbued with a sense of solidity/of sameness and stasis/but nowadays it seems all balance/ fluidity/ movement/ leading with our weighty human heads/ heavy with the presence of absence/ Jelena has lived her whole life alongside this presence/she walks along my left side/sees this weakness as a gift /a source of strength / hah!/"what is seeable, hearable etc. shifts with the interactional space the researcher inhabits, with the time and the purpose in telling, and with the discursive possibilities available (or brought to conscious awareness) at the time of each telling" (Davies, 2000, p. 144) (in)scribing body landscape relations.

It is standard practice for academics to divide their reading / like their thoughts/ into reading for 'the project' and other reading /this is rather like the compartments that hive off "academic prose from poetry, field notes and shopping lists but it became evident during this study that everything I was reading – in the feminist reading group, the newspaper and in the bath – was all slipping around in the mix and providing a source of scaffolding for staring at the park. Thus Kathleen Swift's 'The Morville Hours' which we were reading in the bluestockings became the underpinning for a way of mapping traces left by the Victorian park builders and the BBC Wales (2014) production of 'Under Milkwood' for the centenary of Dylan Thomas's birth led to further readings of other park ghosts. With Mrs. Dai Bread 1 and Mrs. Dai Bread 2 in mind my staring caught traces of ancient people trudging along the coffin paths over to Baddock woods. Indeed, there were any number of contenders in the park most days for the roles of Polly Garter and No Good Boyo. Books blew in as sources by a variety of means, mostly serendipity and a westerly wind

Plateau six

Epilogue/solitude is what I live with a constant lack of/txt

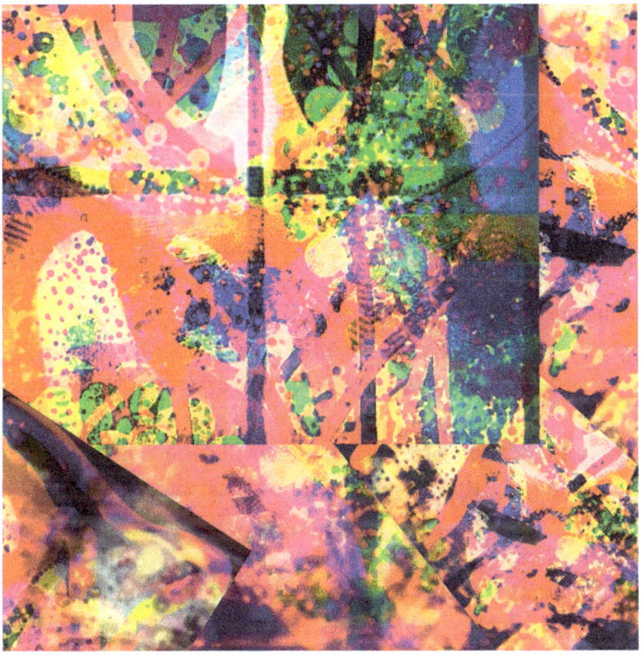

through the window

Starring at the Park: A Poetic Autoethnographic Inquiry, Jane Speedy, 159–176.

SOLITUDE IS WHAT I LIVE WITH A CONSTANT LACK OF/ THE COCKLE-warming/spirit-soothing balms of solitude/I have such craving/ being upstairs 'staring into space' is my nearest equivalent/ just me and the horse chestnut/ our snatched time together firing this craving/

> Words are like nails. You can bang them in like nails and can try to pull them back, as if retrieving them from the wood with the reverse of the hammer, but they always leave holes.
>
> (Anon, 1990, quoted in Rodaway, 2002, p. 1)

in the little bookshop in Westbury Park
I glimpse a title: 'CONTEMPORARY
PHOTOGRAPHY OR WHY THINGS
DON'T HAVE TO BE IN FOCUS' /
this book is speaking to me /

I dreamt again of solitude/of being on my own out on the cliffs in Pembrokeshire/sea sounds/waves against pebbles/gull sounds/ screeches in the wind/alone in the wilds/ I awoke overlooking the park/ surround-sound-scapes of the city/and a space full of secrets/manicured urban secrets/ 115 years of secrets dropped onto paths/buried in unmarked graves and spilling out of bins/ before secrets were inscribed onto paper found floating around in the air after death/now secrets are retrieved from old mobile phones and tablets/ hidden information revealing passwords/ ciphers/ hieroglyphs/ encryptions/
every day as dusk approaches the bearers of secrets come streaming through the park leaving traces/ the park dwellers /yummy mummies/ joggers /dog walkers/drug dealers and circus-school student equivalents of Victorian England (like Clough and Yalom[1] we are going for symbolic equivalents here)/ we see – or almost see – these ghosts (they don't have to be in focus, remember) planting the avenue of lime trees up from the centre and the horse chestnuts around the entrance at the Maurice/ Leopold roads junction/ the new geographical mappers of residual traces tell us about the residual traces of traumatic events/but what of everyday events? /tree plantings/ path sweepings/fence buildings/ what of events so ordinary and lives lived so in

the everyday that their traces go unmapped and their residues untapped?/ the making of a park/like making of the garden at the Morville Dower house[2] / may be etched and scratched and interrupted over (albeit differently) with as many secrets and stories as any site of disturbance and suffering/ you just have to listen for different whispers/there is a six-headed serpent in the park that stalks the paths in the early hours for secrets and stories and scraps of litter/ such intimate geographies

> the changing role of the senses in everyday experiences of space and place. This is a surprisingly neglected geography and one rich in possibilities.
>
> (Rodaway, 2002, p. 3)

SHE HAD OFTEN FLOWN IN HER DREAMS/ SHE HAD BEEN FLYING ALL HER LIFE REALLY/ BUT THIS DREAM SEQUENCE FLYING HARDLY DID JUSTICE TO THE REAL EXPERIENCE/ that moment of flinging herself off the window sill, wings outspread/ that moment of soaring up into the westerly wind/ she never knew quite what to do with her hands and arms and experienced a surfeit of upper body limbs as she crossed them in front of her – the position she had taken up in her primary school nativity play/ a position she had not had to call on in over fifty years/

She was 'awash on a current, a slick of debris, words, papers, scraps, shards, years dispersing itself over darkening waters'... (McCleen, 2013, p. 346) inscribing the park with scraps of text, searching them out of the mouths of other.

Just as Gillian Clarke (2008, pp. 3–8) had dug over Shakespeare's kitchen gardens, finding that in his dream:

'As imagination bodies forth
The form of things unknown, the poet's pen
Turns them to shapes, and gives to airy nothing
A local habitation and a name'

SHE HAD COPIED SCRAPS OF POEMS, PLAYS AND ACADEMIC PAPERS AND CARRYING THEM INTO THE ROOM WITH THE IPAD HAD SAT HERSELF DOWN IN THE BAY WINDOW. Now her stories had given to the airy nothing in the park, dark happenings in the paddling pool and stark, tragic deaths amongst the trees. Forms of things both known and unknown.

> THE BRUTAL, THOUGHTLESS MURDER OF THE MAYOR IN THE PADDLING POOL BY THE WRONGED AND VENGEFUL PROFESSOR IS A SENSELESS ACT undertaken in a shocking, surprising and callous way by the professor of poetic inquiry/the act is out of character; a heat of the moment endeavour, undertaken with, seemingly, no moral or personal responsibility for its consequences, without responsibility to the people of Bristol for murdering their elected mayor/it is an action illustrative of Arendt's unthinking 'banality of evil', not in the sense that the professor was unthinkingly carrying out orders, but in the sense that she was carrying out her crime in a routine, unthinking, uncritical way devoid of responsibility (Butler, 2004) in both moral and criminal content and as a literary form/ The veils between narrator/author/writer/character and reader are at their thinnest during these aspects of the book/as readers we ask ourselves about the relationship between the author (herself a professor) and the professor of poetic inquiry and about the imagined murder mystery and the actual election of a new mayor of Bristol (November 2012) at the time this book was being written/

They did not tell me, on coming out, that everything would seem so loud, would go past me so quickly, that the world would seem so fast. Was this a reaction to being 'institutionalised' or a post-stroke cognitive trope? I was moving as if in a dream, motions slow, spaces gauzy, as if filtered. A poetics of reverie overcame me.

SWALLOWING BRISTOL/ FOG IN THE PARK\PEOPLE COMING OUT OF WHITE BLANK SPACE STARTLING EACH OTHER\GHOST DOGS SNIFFING into cloud bushes/this whole city is living in my world /at first when I came out of hospital/ the city hit me with a barrage of indistinguishable shrouded shapes and noises/ the seagull-pecked, engine-fuelled soundscape merged and swirled on top of a maze of cracked and pockmarked pavements and concrete-coated landscapes/no time or space or earth to breathe between the droning chimes of old George in his tower/at first I had no sense of who was coming at me from the murk or what they had said/were going to say/I was like a provincial peasant at the top of the queue in a fast-food chain/whilst the world fired questions I stared open-mouthed/startled by speed and sound and unfamiliar rhythms/I am now

Oh the poor tired rain, still dripping. A very wet man walks, not quite not skipping…

(Oswald, 2008, p. 583)

accustomed/acculturated/and know where all the holes are in the pavements/ but still cannot discern the sounds directed towards me/this is not a hearing problem/you understand/ more a question of belief/more a serious doubt that this edifice can hold us all up much longer/my particular take on all the gaps and cracks in and beneath the pavements/suggests incoming implosion/a whole aeroplane vanished over the china seas last week/239 people disappeared/ why are we not more surprised?/why not an entire city?/ this morning 428,134 people vanished into the fog/swallowing Bristol/ a provincial city in the south-west of England/ the M4 between Swindon and Cardiff and the M5 between Stroud and Weston-Super-Mare have been closed until further notice/

> Some things are so solid in their reality that one forgets to dream upon their name.
>
> (Bachelard, 1969, p. 30)

WALKING THROUGH THE PARK IN HER NEW 'JACKIE O' STYLE PINK COAT AND HAT WITH HER THICK BLACK TIGHTS AND SHINY PATENT LEATHER SHOES/ SHE QUICKENED HER PACE/ IT WAS A COLD MORNING AND SHE COULD SEE HER OWN WARM BREATH floating in the air before her/ she walked with an audaciously upright posture/leftover from deportment lessons at school/she always wore Chanel number five on workdays/always with the dark pink lipstick/ she looked every inch a lady as she strode out/strode beyond the parameters of this window into a life beyond these borders/

As I look at the park from my window, more than ever, I need 'the power of modern critical theories of how meanings and bodies get made/ not in order to deny meanings and bodies/ but in order to build meanings and bodies that have a chance for life' (Haraway, 1988, p. 580).

LYING JUST BELOW THE PARK'S SURFACE/
FLOAT THE WORD nuggets waiting for distillation/ salient sounds stick in auditory filters/and get caught up in the text-net/ a fine-meshed sound-sieve, sharp eyes and good hearing/these are all the paraphernalia needed for collecting poetic everyday comments in and around the hospital or neighbourhood/ prose is (apparently) okay for academics/ too many words put down where haiku would do?/ poems found lying on the ground/ and trodden into lino corridors/are allowed if we can trace their origins in our sacred data/our holy transcripts/this ritualised cleansing into text of that which is 'empirically' found/ according to Lahman and Richard (2014), citing the sainted Richardson (1993, 2001):

'Lousy poetry
masquerades
as research
and vice versa'

yet this whole murder inquiry/ ethnography/ life-story malarkey is nothing but a performance/ masquerade/ show me the text that masquerades as nothing and I'll give you back thin air /or the instructions for setting the timer on your boiler and the shopping list he dropped on the landing/ (he forgot the toothpaste) / these scraps could enter the holy transcripts yet as 'field notes?' / 'landing notes?'/ 'selected pages collected in the researcher's journal?'/ 'filtered /annotated litter?'/ I like the sound of 'vice-versa' (above) / lousy poetry or lousy practices of inquiry? /

I am very attuned, these days, to my body/myself in a state of becoming/ always becoming never there/being/ becoming lousy/everything changing/ I am with Gale (2014, p. 1), who finds this a space or domain of' 'implication and inference, suggestion and nuance, sense and intuition' I recall the word embodiment as if it was imbued with a sense of solidity/of sameness and stasis/but nowadays it seems all balance/ fluidity/ movement/ leading with our weighty human heads/ heavy with the presence of absence/ Jelena has lived her whole life alongside this presence/she walks along my left side/sees this weakness as a gift /a source of strength / hah!/

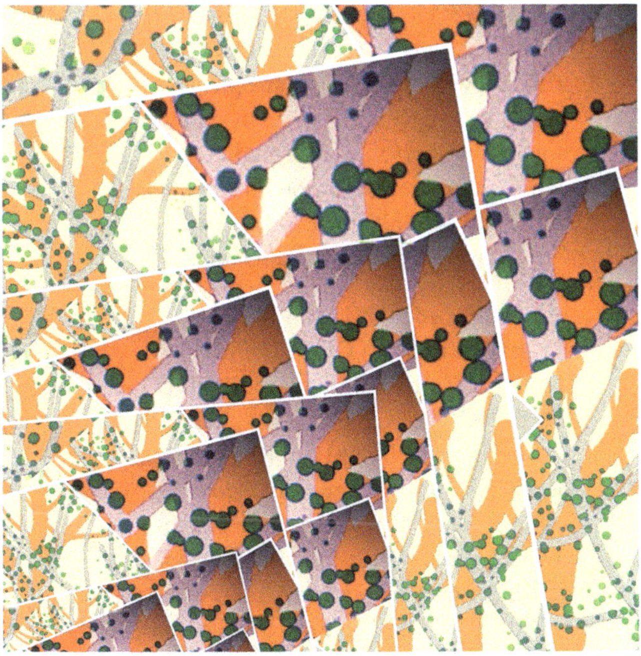

fragmented views

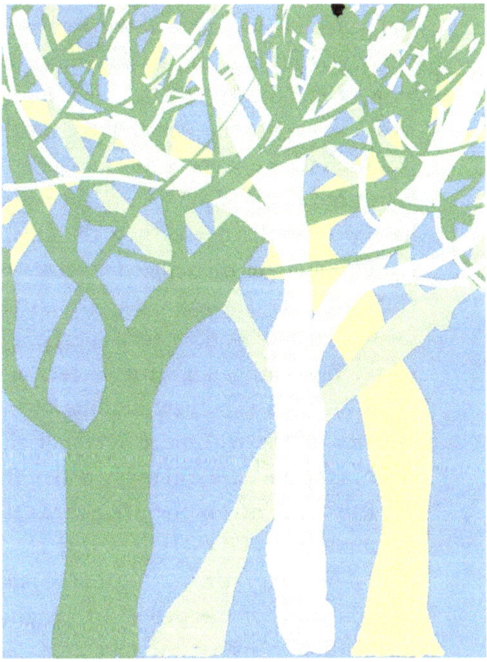

early morning in the park

"what is seeable, hearable etc. shifts with
the interactional space the researcher
inhabits, with the time and the purpose
in telling, and with the discursive
possibilities available (or brought to
conscious awareness) at the time of each
telling" (Davies, 2000, p. 144)
(in)scribing body landscape relations,

WE ARE LEFT WITH PLENTY OF UNANSWERED QUESTIONS AT THE END /IF THIS IS THE END/ THE HORSE CHESTNUT TREES WOULD HAVE SAID NOTHING/ despite the heavy-handed interrogation tactics of the police/the avenue of plane trees were really lime trees/ and the joggers had not witnessed anything, which still does not explain how the peacock feather pattern from the Kantha shawl was launched as a pair of wings from a window sill/ and the notion that 'the winged creature of Bristol' the south-west's answer to the 'Angel of the north' was too much of a freak role for the professor of poetic inquiry to take on/nor have we ever discovered how the mayor found out about the winged creature or what pressures he brought to bear/they say he had it all worked out as part of his marketing campaign/ the detectives, especially Scossi, /knew nothing of the identity of the real murderer/ but the trees in the park are still dying and nothing can be done for them/here we are all implicated and every morning clock time stands very still waiting for the park to wake and for the people to imagine their everyday lives into movement and light/we are left with all plots unravelling and scattering to the westerly wind/ having barely scratched the surface of 'those features of the human realm that go beyond linearity, that involve movement not only from past to present but present to past' (Freeman, 2010, p. 178) we are still waiting for the prequel to everyday lives and narrative imagination (Andrews, 2014) everyday imagination and narrative lives.

It is hard perhaps for you to imagine these conversations drifting across the park/snatches caught in the roots of trees/the big hollows of the copper beech down by the west entrance/ I see the person and do not hear them in the conventional sense/ but I am listening/ have been tuned into them for days/ weeks/months/as they move across the space of the park/ The shared eye. A multiplicity of 'I's/You pass the paper across/I-dentity moves from you to me to them to us/authorship evaporates, ownership collapses – the soft contract hardens in the sun like terracotta/the writing takes the lead, the writing writes us, the writing writes our lives, the agency of objects plays us for patsies/inhabited silences between collaborative 'I's /we have our celebrities/the sainted Massey and the oft- quoted Ingold /we've got ourselves entangled with the aftershock of the blessed Barad / these are the post-post structuralist patron saints of

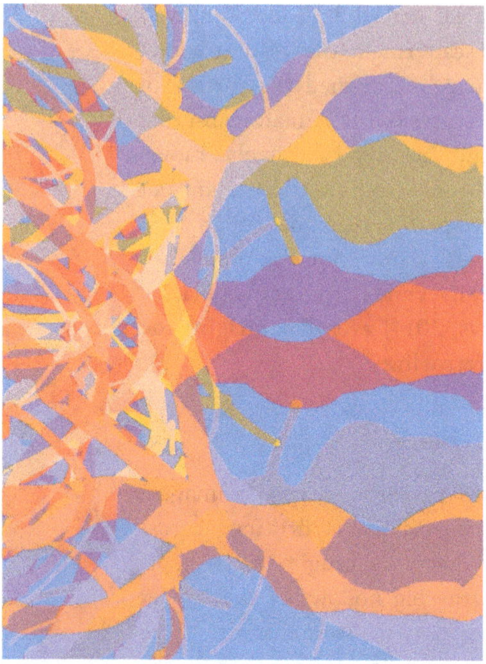

paths remember people

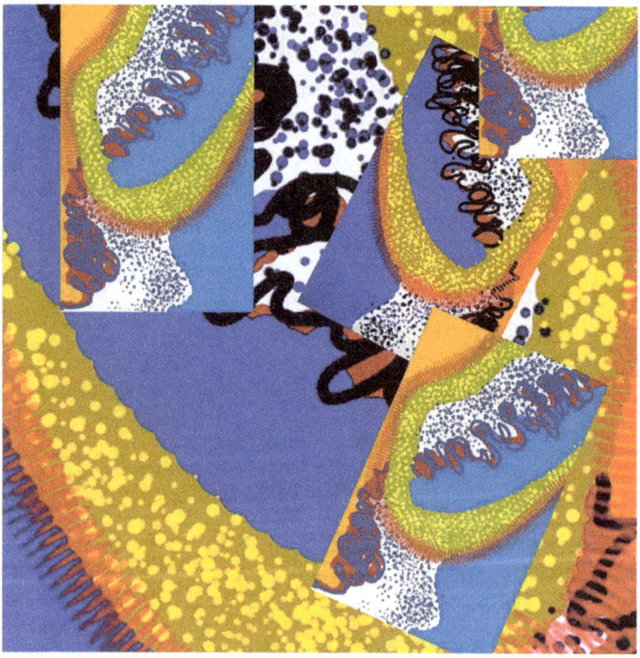

splintered
pathway

the new geographies and physics – we are alone at the shrine/we have new Gods we worship neither Zeus, nor Jehovah nor bask in the mirror of our shared humanity/ Om meaho rengay kyo/ Om myaho ren gay kyo/ shanti, shanti, shanti/

sitting in the sun on the deck my wings spread out behind me to dry – I felt glorious – people's lives criss-crossing/ memories blowing the leaves/ winter waste bag collection/ screaming at Sarah/practices of love/parking and driving/the gym/the exercise class/ the bank/going to my art class for a love affair with Indian ink/looking at Christmas trees/the house with the picture of Lenin/the house where they filmed 'Casualty'/ meory and geography/ the church/going to St David's/

A shadow of the self I might have been becoming, overlooked/ I overlook the park/ the woman in the mirror carrying the peacock's eye wings says her life is fine/ just not how she imagined it to be/ breaking the mirror into shards and fragments takes seven years to heal/ soul healing halts the gaze behind the eyes that you see in mirrors/ clicks again in our dreams/grey snakes on the beach/ or was it driftwood?/ my life all folded neatly never happened/the life they opened up after we had all gone surprised them and left them lightheaded and giddy with stolen and shocking stories/we put the neatly stacked lives away in the cupboard for later/ they would leave no traces if lived now/ this rich residue would drench everyone who demonstrated a glimmer of interest/breaking mirrors hung with shawls and scarves opens the souls of those who died in the room/ ghost reflections shattered/ Miss Jenner the milliner lived here before us in the house her father built/ the mirror breakage releases old ghosts/

> My life all folded neatly never happened/the life they opened up after we had all gone surprised them/

you leave me sitting in the sun outside the Sloop and go off on my favourite walk/ 'will you be alright?' you ask/yes of course I say/what will you do you ask/write a poem I say/ will that be alright you say/ yes of course I reply /I sip my red wine/ as you all get your gear on/and then as soon as you leave/my battery runs out and I am left with nothing to write on or with/ I sit in the sun and stare across the harbour at the cloud shadows skidding across the warm brick walls of the ruins on the other side/there is a wind out on the Irish sea/ but here in the pub garden/ in the little inlet /we are sheltered/ I close my eyes and think of you/in my mind's eye we are never 2 old ladies hobbling down the quayside/but young women striding out with far too much/ far too curly hair for our own good heads held high, hands held tight/

the day the mayor's mother came to look at the paddling pool/windswept and distraught/she stood too near the edge/'surviving your adult children puts you out of synch with your own future' she said/ we had weather that day/the trees creaked in the 80 mile an hour wind/ none fell/she walked between 2 policemen/she carried her havoc in her face and hands/I watched from my bedroom eyrie/

there's a bloke texting in the park/ it's Arthur – no it isn't – /he's as tall as Arthur nearly – /and not looking where he's walking /ambling along texting like a kid he looks about sixty/maybe more/ smart phones/ stupid people /

they don't take provincial cripples in the London Borough of Westminster – our blue badges count for nothing there/ I suppose somebody at head office had a bad but statistically accurate dream one day that all the 'out of town cripples' in the European Union came on the same day and /parking on all the double yellow lines / clogged up the traffic in their already congested city/crippling congestion/

THE OPEN SPACE OF THE PARK INVITES DETOURS FROM THE TRAMLINES OF PEOPLE'S LIVES / IN THE SUNSHINE PEOPLE FEEL COMPELLED TO STRAY FROM THE PATH/NO TRAFFIC – ONLY KIDS ON BIKES and skateboards/ there is a freedom to make new paths/ divergent and random tracks appear in

the summer and smudge across the grass adding to the criss-crossed concrete hatchings and dainty fox-ways/short cuts across corners and also inexplicably lengthy and meandering detours/the pace of the park differs from that of the surrounding streets/there is skipping and running/loping and bounding/in the rain the park invites speed and in the sunshine idleness/
in the streets the pace is uniform/ turgid/greyer/

> Individuals emerge through and as part of their entangled inter-relating.
>
> (Barad, 2003)

This text is often hidden between the tramlines of its own borders/ you have to seek it out/ in places it is almost lost/there is not much open space/I anticipate detours and have left margins for comments if so desired/what if/ in thirty years/ a copy comes to light and all the margins are pristine white/ what then? /I anticipate the skipping of whole chunks/just as I have skipped great swathes in the writing, so shall you in the reading/we are making it up together/

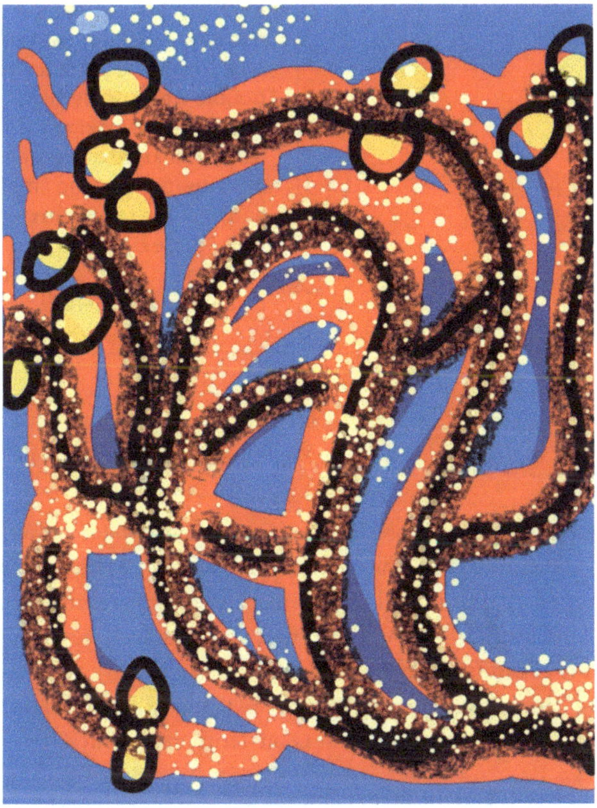

six-headed serpent

> Over here more is inscribed on the margins of the park than can usually be seen amidst the footfalls/slushy ground/scattered body parts between the trees/
> two old mattresses lean against the pine tree at the entrance/remains of a double wedding perhaps? /the trees stand silently/making their inside leaves/the gaze of the trees is not obvious /until you go amongst them and hear the rustle turn to you as you walk/ these borderlands are neither pencilled in nor blank/holding anxiety by the hand/in silence/

In attempting to write/produce and curate this book it has written/produced and curated me. The narrative incoherence of life following a stroke has opened up the entangled gossamer threads of life (mine and those of other life forms/other lives lived) that underlay and overlay traditional accounts of carefully separated lives lived in narrative coherence. In my writing I am not spread evenly between plateaux, but rather, some territories take longer than others to cross. I constantly repeat myself.

This book is not an intimate personal narrative, but rather a distanced, ethical account that both winds its way across and troubles various times and spaces. There is, as Freeman (1998) would concur, a distance and a difference between chronological and autobiographical time, and I hope I have conveyed that distance and some of those differences to readers of this book. Nevertheless, I have felt compelled to give this account as I stare out into the horse chestnut trees and they stare back. Somewhere along the gossamer threads of entanglement, co-produced in this mutual gaze, my humanity is lost in a thicket of treeness, just as the treeness of the horse chestnut is lost in its humanity.

Notes

First plateau

1. Riessman, C (2004).
2. 'Dropbox': a web-based file sharing system; www.dropbox.com/
3. Freeman, M (2010).
4. Five rhythms dancing: a therapeutic dance practice, created by Gabrielle Roth (1989).
5. Three 20th/21st century stroke survival stories written in differently culturally positioned but nonetheless coherent , typically triumphalist 'western illness' narrative style: Bolte-Taylor, J (2009), Klein, B (1997) and McCrum, R (1998). McCrum's is a more literary text and Bolte-Taylor's contains more of the requisite neuro-science, but all three of these texts follow the same coherent narrative model of triumph over illness, narrowly outwitting death.
6. Marr, A (2013).
7. Moss, S (2014): review of Finkel, I (2014).

Second plateau

1. Ann Carson's two volumes of poetry, 'Autobiography of Red' (1999) and its sequel, 'Red doc>' (2013), trace the 3,000-year-old story of the creature Geryon (later known as G).
2. Emily Dickinson's poem, 'Tell all the Truth but tell it slant', leaves the truth to 'dazzle gradually'.

Third plateau

1. See www.leedsmet.ac.uk/research/professor-andrew-sparkes.htm

Fifth plateau

1. Martha Nussbaum (1999) wrote a famously vicious critique of her fellow-feminist philosopher Judith Butler and the language she used, arguing that Butler's work was entirely theoretical and was not connected with the real lives of women.
2. Patti Lather and Chris Smithies' book, *Troubling the Angels: Women Living with HIV/AIDS*, to which this current text owes a debt in that it was a precursor that troubled traditional academic layout conventions, was not the book the participants in the project wanted.

Sixth plateau

1. See Clough, P (2002) and Yalom, I (1989).
2. See Swift, K (2008).

References

Literature

Adkins, B (2012) Deleuze and Badiou on the nature of events, in: *Philosophy Compass*, 7 (8) 507–516.

Aitken, W (2004) Anne Carson: The art of poetry, in: *Paris Review*, 88 (fall), 171.

Andrews, M (2014) *Narrative imagination and everyday life*, Oxford: Oxford University Press.

Austen, J (1814/2013) *Mansfield park*, Derry, UK: Callender Press.

Bachelard, G (1971) *The poetics of reverie*, Boston: Beacon Press.

Bachelard, G (1994) *The poetics of space*, Boston: Beacon Press.

Barad (2003) Posthumanist performativity: Towards an understanding of how matter comes to matter, in: *Signs: Journal of Women, in Culture and Society*, 28 (3) 801–830.

Barad, K (2007) *Meeting the universe halfway, Quantum physics and the entanglement of matter and meaning*, Durham, NC: Duke University Press.

Benjamin, W (1927/1999) *The Arcades Project*, Cambridge, MA: Harvard University Press.

Berger, J (1967/2008) *Ways of seeing*, Harmondsworth, UK: Penguin Modern Classics.

Bogue, R (2003) *Deleuze on music, painting and the arts*, London: Routledge.

Bolte-Taylor, J. (2009) *My stroke of insight*, London: Hodder and Stoughton.

Bowers, M (2004) *Magic(al) realism: (The new critical idiom)*, London: Routledge.

Buchan, K (2014) Decelerator helmet: Viewing the world in slow motion, in: *Guardian*, July 10.

Butler, J (2004) *Precarious life: The powers of mourning and violence*, New York: Verso.

Carruthers, M. (2008) (2nd ed) *The book of memory: Memory in medieval culture*, Cambridge, UK: Cambridge University Press.

Carson, A (1992) *Glass, irony and God*, New York: New Directions.

Carson, A (1999) *Autobiography of red*, London: Cape Poetry.

Carson, A (2003) *If not, winter: Fragments of Sappho*, London: Virago.

Carson, A (2013) *Red doc>*, London: Cape Poetry.

Cixous, H and Calle-Gruber, M (1997) *Rootprints: Memory and life-writing*, London: Routledge.

Clandinin, J (2008) cited in: Clandinin, J and Cave, M (2008) Creating pedagogical spaces for developing doctor professional identity, in: *Medical Education* 42 (8) 765–770.

Clandinin, J and Connelly, M (2004) *Narrative inquiry: Experience and story in qualitative research (education)*, San Francisco: Jossey Bass.

Clarke, G (2011) *Collected poems*, Manchester, UK: Carcanet Press.

Clarke, G (2008) *At the source: A writer's year*, Manchester, UK: Carcanet Press.

Clarke, G (2011) *Collected poems*, Manchester, UK. Carcanet Press.

Clough, P. (2002) *Narratives and fictions in educational research (Doing qualitative research in educational settings)*, Maidenhead, UK: Open University Press.

Csikszentmihalyi, M (2002) *Flow: The psychology of optimal experience*, New York: Harper Collins.

Davies, B (2000) *(In)scribing body/landscape relations*, Walnut Creek, CA: AltaMira Press.

Davies, B and Gannon, S (2013) Collective biography and the entangled enlivening of being, in: *International Review of Qualitative Research* 5(4) 357–376.

Deleuze, G, and Guattari, F (1987) *A thousand plateaus: Capitalism and schizophrenia* (B. Massumi, Trans.), Minneapolis: University of Minnesota Press.

Denzin, N (1997) *Interpretive ethnography*, Thousand Oaks, CA: Sage.

Derrida, J (1981) *Positions*, Chicago: University of Chicago Press.

Dickinson, E (1976) Tell all the truth, in: *Complete poems*, London: Faber and Faber.

Duffy, C A (2010) *Feminine gospels*, London: Picador.

Duffy, C A (2011) *The bees*, London: Picador.

Ebenstein (2006) Towards an archetypal psychology of disability based on the Hyphaestus myth, in: *Disability Studies Quarterly*, 26 (4). www.dsq-sds.org

Eco, U (2004) *Mouse or rat? Translation as negotiation*, London: Orion Books.

Eggers, D (2000) *A heartbreaking work of staggering genius*, New York: Simon and Schuster.

Etherington, K (2004) *Becoming a reflexive researcher, using our selves in research*, London: Jessica Kingsley.

Faris, W (2004) *Ordinary enchantments: Magical realism and the remystification of narrative*, Nashville, TN: Vanderbilt University Press.

Finkel, I (2007) *The last resort library*, Glasgow: Kennedy and Boyd.

Finkel, I (2014) *The ark before Noah: Decoding the story of the flood*, London: Hodder and Stoughton.

Freeman, M (1998) Mythical time, historical time and the narrative fabric of the self, in: *Narrative Inquiry*, 8 (1) 27–50.

Freeman, M (2010) *Hindsight: The promise and peril of looking backward*, Oxford, UK: Oxford University Press.

Gale, K (2014) Moods, tones, flavours: Living with intensities as inquiry, in: *Qualitative Inquiry*, January, 1–7.

Garland-Thomson, R (2005) Staring at the other, in: *Disability Studies Quarterly* 25 (4) www.dsq-sds.org/

Garland-Thomson, R (2009) *Staring: How we look*, Oxford, UK: Oxford University Press.

Gauntlett, D (2011) *Making is connecting, the social meaning of creativity from D.I.Y. and knitting to YouTube and web 2.0*, Cambridge, UK: Polity Press.

Geertz, C (1977) *The interpretation of cultures*, New York, Basic Books.

Greene, M (1995). *Releasing the imagination: Essays on education, the arts, and social change*. San Francisco: Jossey-Bass.

Haraway, D (1988) Situated knowledges: The science question, in: feminism and the privilege of partial perspective, in: *Feminist Studies*, 14 (3) 575–599.

Hein, S (2013) Thinking and writing with ontological time in qualitative inquiry, in: *Qualitative Inquiry* 19 (7) 493–501.

Ingold, T. (2007) *Lines: A brief history*, London: Routledge.

Jackson, A and Mazzei, L (2013) Plugging one text into another: Thinking with theory in qualitative research, in: *Qualitative Inquiry* 19 261–271.

James, W (1890/2013) *The principles of psychology*, New York: Cosimo Classics.
Joyce, J (1922/2008) *Ulysses*, Oxford, UK: Oxford's World Classics.

Keats, J note on copy of 'Paradise lost' cited in Carson, A (2002, p. 186) *The beauty of the husband: A fictional essay in 29 Tangos*, London: Cape Poetry.
King, N (2000) *Memory, narrative, identity: Remembering the self*, Edinburgh: Edinburgh University Press.
Klee, P (1920) *Creative confessions*, London: Tate.
Klein, B (1998) *Slow dance: A story of stroke, love and disability*, Berkeley, CA: Wildcat Canyon Press.

Lahman, M and Richard, V (2014) Appropriated poetry: Archival poetry in research, in: *Qualitative Inquiry*, 20 (3) 344–355.
Lather, P (2007) *Getting lost: Feminist efforts towards a doubled science*, New York: SUNY.

Macfarlane, R (2012) *The old ways: A journey on foot*, London: Hamish Hamilton.
Macfarlane, R, Richards, D and Donwood, S (2013) *Holloway*, London: Faber and Faber.
Marr, A (2013) *A short book about drawing*, London: Quadrille.
Massey, D (2000) *For space*, Thousand Oaks, CA: Sage.
Mazzei (2007) *Inhabited silences in qualitative research: Putting poststructural theory to work*, New York: Peter Lang.
McCleen, G (2013) *The professor of poetry*, London: Spectre.
McCrum, R (1998) *My year off: Re-discovering life after a stroke*, London: Picador.
Morrison, T (1987/2007) *Beloved*, New York: Vintage Classics.
Moss, S (2014) Noah's Ark was round so the ancient tablets tell us: Review of Finkel, I (2014), *The ark before Noah: Decoding the story of the flood, London*: Hodder and Stoughton, in: *Guardian* February 11.
Myerhoff (1982) Introduction in Ruby, J (Ed) *The crack in the mirror: Reflexive perspectives in anthropology*, Philadelphia, University of Pennsylvania Press.

Nussbaum, M (1999) The professor of parody, in: *New Republic Online*.

Orwell, G ([1945]2003) *Animal farm*, Harmondsworth, UK: Penguin Books.
Oswald, A (2008) *Woods, etc.* London: Faber and Faber.

Piirto, J (2009) The question of quality and qualifications: Writing inferior poems as qualitative research, in: *Qualitative Studies in Education*, 15 (4) 431–445.
Plath, S (1963/2005) *The bell jar*, London: Faber and Faber.
Prendergast, M (2009) The phenomena of poetry in research, Poem is what? Poetic Inquiry in qualitative social science research, in: Prendergast, M, Leggo, C and Sameshima, P (2009) (Eds.) *Poetic inquiry*, Rotterdam: Sense.
Prendergast, M, Leggo, C and Sameshima, P (2009) (Eds.) *Poetic inquiry*, Rotterdam: Sense.
Pullman, P (2003) *Lyra's oxford*, New York: Knopf

Reece, J (2015/forthcoming) *Losing the plot: A fictional exploration into Narrative Inquiry*, University of Bristol: unpublished doctoral thesis.
Richardson, L (1997) The poetic representation of lives, in *Fields of play, constructing an academic life*, New Brunswick, NJ: Rutgers University Press.
Richardson, L (1993). Poetics, dramatics, and transgressive validity: The case of the skipped line, in: *Sociological Quarterly*, 34, 695–710.
Richardson, L (2001) Poetic representation of interviews in Gubrium, J and Holsteien, J (Eds.) *Handbook of interview research*, Thousand Oaks, CA: Sage.

Riessman, C (2004) A thrice told tale: New readings of an old story, in: Hurwitz, B, Greenhagh, P, and Skultans, V, (2004) *Narrative research in health and illness,* Chichester, UK: Wiley.

Riessman, C (2008) *Narrative methods for the human sciences,* Thousand Oaks, CA: Sage.

Rodaway, P (2002) *Sensuous geographies: Body, sense and place,* London: Routledge.

Ronai, C R (1995) Multiple reflections of child sex abuse: An argument for a layered account, in: *Journal of Contemporary Ethnography* 23 395–426.

Roth, G (1989) *Maps to ecstasy,* Novato, CA: New World.

Ruby, J (2000) *Picturing culture: Explorations of film and anthropology,* Chicago: University of Chicago Press.

Rushdie, S (1980) *Midnight's children,* New York: Vintage.

Sakellariadis, A, Chromy, S, Martin, V, Speedy, J, Trahar, S, Williams, S, and Wilson, S (2008) Friend and foe: Technology in a collaborative writing group, in: *Qualitative Inquiry* 14 1205–1222.

Sameshima, P (2007) *Seeing red – a pedagogy of parallax: An epistolatory bildingsroman on artful scholarly inquiry,* Amherst, NY: Cambria Press.

Solnit, R (2005) *A field guide to getting lost,* London, Viking.

Speedy, J. (2008) *Narrative inquiry and psychotherapy,* Hound Mills, UK: Palgrave/Macmillan.

Speedy, J with Margie, Fay, Jack and Pauline Jones (2005) Failing to come to terms with things: A multistoried conversation about poststructuralist ideas and narrative practices in response to some of life's failures, in: *Counselling and Psychotherapy Research* 5 (1) 65–74.

Springgay, S, Irwin, R and Kind, S (2005) A/r/tography as living inquiry through art and text, in: *Qualitative Inquiry* 11 897–912.

Swift, K (2008) *The Morville Hours: The story of a garden,* London: Bloomsbury.

Thomas, D (1954/2003) *Under milk wood,* Phoenix, AZ: Phoenix.

Till, K (Ed.) (2010) *Mapping spectral places,* brochure for exhibit, Virginia Tech.

Tomalin (2012) *Charles Dickens: A life,* Harmondsworth, UK: Penguin.

Transtroemer, T (1997/2011) *New collected poems,* Newcastle Upon Tyne, UK: Bloodaxe Books

Weems, M (2003) *Public education and the imagination-intellect: I speak from the wound in my mouth,* New York: Peter Lang.

West, D (2012) *Signs of hope: Deaf-hearing family life,* Newcastle upon Tyne, UK: Cambridge Scholars Press.

White, M (2004) *Narrative practice and exotic lives:Resurrecting diversity in everyday life.* Adelaide, South Australia: Dulwich Centre.

Winterson, J (2004) *Lighthousekeeping,* London: Harper Perrenial.

Woolf, V (1925/1996) *Mrs. Dalloway,* Boston: Wordsworth Classics.

Woolf, V (2002) (Eds: Shulkind, J and Lee, H) *Moments of being: Autobiographical writings,* London: Pimlico.

Yalom, I (1989) *Love's executioner,* New York: Basic Books.

Other media

Astley, N (2011) *Transtroemer receives the Nobel prize for literature:* www.youtube.com/watch?v=28Uo61rvUms

BBC Wales (2014) *Under Milkwood,* www.bbc.co.uk/programmes/galleries/p01y7cxc

Bauby, J (2008) *The diving bell and the butterfly,* New York, Harper Perrenial.

Bourdieu, P (1990) Homo Academicus, Redwood City, CA: Stanford University Press.

Buchan, K (2014) Decelerator helmet: Viewing the world in slow motion, in: *Guardian/Observer Technology Monthly* www.theguardian.com/technology/2014/jul/10/decelerator-helmet-lorenz potthast-slow-motion

Fellowes, J (2010–present) *Downton Abbey* www.itv.com/downtonabbey

Friends of St Andrews Park website: friendsofstandrewspark.ning.com/

Haneke, M. (Dir.) (2012) *'Amour',* Artificial Eye Films: London.

Hockney, D (2012) *A bigger picture,* www.imdb.com/title/tt1768919/

Leslie, E, *The Benjamin papers,* from Militant Esthetix: www.militantesthetic.co.uk

Lindemann, K. (2013) Listening for echoes: Hypertext, performativity and online narratives of grief, in*: Liminalities, a Journal of Performance Studies* 9 (2) liminalities.net/9-2/lindemann.pdf

McCarthy, T (Dir.) *The Visitor,* Halcyon Pictures.

Nobbs, K (2011) *Fragments of silence,* an unbound single edition book, from: www.katenobbs.com/

Riessman, C (2004)). A thrice told tale: New readings of an old story, in: Hurwitz, B, Greenhagh, P and Skultans, V (2004) *Narrative research in health and illness,* Chichester, UK: Wiley.

Roth, G (1989) *Maps to ecstacy,* Novato, CA: New World.

Ruby, J (2006) *Maintaining diversity: An ethnographic study of Oak Park, Illinois* astro.temple.edu/~ruby/opp/

Till , K (2010) Mapping spectral traces, *www.research.spia.vt.edu/events/spectral-traces/*

Warnock, M (2012) *Parliament's moral duty on assisted dying* www.theguardian.com/commentisfree/2012/jan/01/mary-warnock-assisted-suicide

Winehouse, A (2006) 'Rehab' from *'Back to black',* Island Records, London: www.youtube.com/watch?v=TJAfLE39ZZ8

About the author

Prolific scholar **Jane Speedy** maintains an international reputation for developing innovative interdisciplinary qualitative research methodologies. Professor Emeritus in the Graduate School of Education at the University of Bristol, she teaches narrative inquiry and other research methods at the intersection of arts and social sciences. Her current focus is on collaborative writing and various forms of collaborative text production, including collective biography, writing as inquiry, and juxtapositions of various visual and written textual forms. She has a particular interest in web 2.0 technologies, such as blogs, wikis, and Twitter as sites for radical collaborations. Jane was also the coordinator of the Narrative Inquiry Centre in the School of Education at the University of Bristol. She is author of *Narrative Inquiry and Psychotherapy* and co-editor of *Collaborative Writing as Inquiry*.

For Product Safety Concerns and Information please contact our EU representative GPSR@taylorandfrancis.com
Taylor & Francis Verlag GmbH, Kaufingerstraße 24, 80331 München, Germany

www.ingramcontent.com/pod-product-compliance
Lightning Source LLC
LaVergne TN
LVHW011133300926
849160LV00008B/633

* 9 7 8 1 6 2 9 5 8 1 2 3 1 *